‖‖‖ ‖ ‖‖‖‖‖‖ ‖‖ ‖ ‖‖ ‖‖‖‖‖‖ ‖‖‖‖‖‖‖‖ ‖‖ ‖‖‖

☞ W9-CFO-437

Evaluation and Management of Early HIV Infection

Early HIV Infection
Guideline Panel

Wafaa El-Sadr, MD, MPH, Co-Chair
James M. Oleske, MD, MPH, Co-Chair
Bruce D. Agins, MD
Kay A. Bauman, MD, MPH
Carol L. Brosgart, MD
Gina M. Brown, MD
Jaime V. Geaga, PA-C, MPH
Deborah Greenspan, BDS, DSc, ScD
Karen Hein, MD, BMS
William L. Holzemer, RN, PhD
Rudolph E. Jackson, MD
Michael K. Lindsay, MD, MPH
Harvey J. Makadon, MD
Martha W. Moon, MS, RN
Claire A. Rappoport, MS
Gwendolyn Scott, MD
Walter W. Shervington, MD
Lawrence C. Shulman, ACSW
Constance B. Wofsy, MD, MA

U.S. Department of Health and Human Services
Public Health Service
Agency for Health Care Policy and Research

AHCPR Publication No. 94-0572
January 1994

Guideline Development and Use

Guidelines are systematically developed statements to assist practitioner and patient decisions about appropriate health care for specific clinical conditions. This guideline was developed by a multidisciplinary panel of private-sector clinicians and other experts convened by the Agency for Health Care Policy and Research (AHCPR). The panel employed an explicit, science-based methodology and expert clinical judgment to develop specific statements on patient assessment and management for the clinical condition selected.

Extensive literature searches were conducted, and critical reviews and syntheses were used to evaluate empirical evidence and significant outcomes. Peer review and field review were undertaken to evaluate the validity, reliability, and utility of the guideline in clinical practice. The panel's recommendations are primarily based on the published scientific literature. When the scientific literature was incomplete or inconsistent in a particular area, the recommendations reflect the professional judgment of panel members and consultants. In some instances, there was not unanimity of opinion.

The guideline reflects the state of knowledge, current at the time of publication, on effective and appropriate care. Given the inevitable changes in the state of scientific information and technology, periodic review, updating, and revision will be done. We believe that the AHCPR-assisted clinical guideline development process will make positive contributions to the quality of care in the United States. We encourage practitioners and patients to use the information provided in this clinical practice guideline. The recommendations may not be appropriate for use in all circumstances. Decisions to adopt any particular recommendation must be made by the practitioner in light of available resources and circumstances presented by individual patients.

> J. Jarrett Clinton, MD
> *Administrator*
> *Agency for Health Care Policy and Research*

Publication of this guideline does not necessarily represent endorsement by the U.S. Department of Health and Human Services.

Foreword

According to the World Health Organization, between 30 and 40 million men, women, and children around the world will be infected with the human immunodeficiency virus (HIV) by the year 2000. Others have estimated that this number may be as high as 110 million. By the turn of the century, acquired immunodeficiency syndrome (AIDS) will be the third most common cause of death in the United States. This growing presence of HIV necessitates that primary care providers become involved in and knowledgeable about HIV care. The growing population of individuals and their families living with HIV also need guidance in seeking and accessing appropriate care.

This guideline provides such recommendations for health care providers and people living with HIV. Philosophically, it recognizes the unique character of the HIV epidemic and the need for a close partnership of providers and consumers. The expert panel that prepared the guideline included representation from both groups in its membership and among the peer reviewers.

Because appropriate assessment and treatment during the initial phase of the infection can have great impact on an individual's quality of life, the panel focused on specific aspects of evaluating and managing early HIV infection. Also included are discussion and recommendations relating to non-medical issues which are intimately related to HIV care.

Thus, the panel's challenge was to include specific medical care approaches for the provider within the broader social and psychological concerns of the patient. This document provides recommendations for a wide range of issues, including immunologic monitoring, specific treatments for HIV infection and commonly associated infections such as tuberculosis and syphilis, issues affecting special groups (such as women, children, and adolescents), case management, and health care policy. It should be noted that the guideline does not address many other areas important to early HIV care.

The past decade has seen many changes in the management of individuals living with HIV infection. The pace of advances in HIV care will make it imperative to update this guideline continually. Although there remain many issues that this panel has not addressed (these are enumerated throughout the guideline), the guideline provides a model for addressing issues of importance to individuals and families living with HIV.

Early HIV Infection Guideline Panel

Abstract

This guideline is a manual of selected protocols for the evaluation and management of the initial stage of infection caused by the human immunodeficiency virus (HIV). It consists of the recommendations of a national, private-sector panel of physicians, dentists, nurses, nurse practitioners, physician assistants, social workers, and medical consumers. These recommendations were made as a result of an exhaustive search and analysis of relevant literature and the extensive clinical experience and expertise of panel participants. Whenever possible, the recommendations were based on an evaluation of published evidence. When scientific evidence was inadequate, panel consensus was used as the basis for recommendations. Each recommendation is followed by a rating that indicates the degree to which it is evidence based. Public testimony, peer review, and a feasibility review were also part of the guideline's development process.

Key topics addressed in the guideline include: antiretroviral therapy and disclosure of HIV status; monitoring of CD4 cell counts and initiation of PCP prophylaxis; testing and preventive therapy for tuberculosis and syphilis; conduct and timing of oral examination, eye examination, and Papanicolaou smear assessment; pregnancy counseling; care for adolescents with HIV infection; evaluation and management of early HIV infection in infants and children; case management for persons living with HIV; and access and availability of care. It should be noted that the guideline does not represent a comprehensive guide to early HIV care; rather, it details only selected aspects of such care.

El-Sadr W, Oleske JM, Agins BD et al. *Evaluation and Management of Early HIV Infection. Clinical Practice Guideline No. 7.* AHCPR Publication No. 94-0572. Rockville, MD: Agency for Health Care Policy and Research, Public Health Service, U.S. Department of Health and Human Services, January 1994.

Panel Members

Wafaa El-Sadr, MD, MPH
Panel Co-chair
Associate Professor of
Clinical Medicine
Columbia University
Chief, Division of Infectious
Diseases
Harlem Hospital Center

James M. Oleske, MD, MPH
Panel Co-chair
Francois-Xavier Bagnoud
Professor of Pediatrics
Director, Division of Allergy,
Immunology, and Infectious
Diseases
New Jersey Medical School

Bruce D. Agins, MD
Assistant Medical Director,
AIDS Institute
NY State Department of Health

Kay A. Bauman, MD, MPH
John A. Burns School of Medicine
Wahiawa General Hospital

Carol L. Brosgart, MD
Medical Director
East Bay AIDS Center
Alta Bates Medical Center

Gina M. Brown, MD
Department of Obstetrics and
Gynecology
Columbia Presbyterian
Medical Center

Jaime V. Geaga, PA-C, MPH
Filipino Task Force on AIDS

**Deborah Greenspan,
BDS, DSc, ScD**
Clinical Professor
Division of Oral Medicine
University of California,
San Francisco

Karen Hein, MD, BMS
Professor, Department of Pediatrics
Director, Adolescent AIDS Program
Albert Einstein College of Medicine

**William L. Holzemer,
RN, PhD**
Professor and Associate Dean for
Research
University of California,
San Francisco

Rudolph E. Jackson, MD
Professor of Pediatrics
Morehouse School of Medicine

Michael K. Lindsay, MD, MPH
Associate Professor
Grady Memorial Hospital

Harvey J. Makadon, MD
Assistant Professor of Medicine
Harvard Medical School

Martha W. Moon, MS, RN
Nurse Practitioner

Claire A. Rappoport, MS
San Francisco Area AIDS
Education and Training Center
San Francisco General Hospital

Gwendolyn Scott, MD
Professor, Department of Pediatrics
University of Miami
School of Medicine

Walter W. Shervington, MD
Division of Mental Health
Office of Human Services
Baton Rouge, LA

Lawrence C. Shulman, MSW, ACSW
Sociomedical Resource Associates

Constance B. Wofsy, MD, MA
Professor of Clinical Medicine
University of California,
San Francisco

Acknowledgments

It was the best of times, it was the worst of times, it was the age
of wisdom, it was the age of foolishness, it was the epic of belief,
it was the epic of incredulity, it was the season of Light, it was the
season of Darkness, it was the spring of hope, it was the winter
of despair...

Charles Dickens, *A Tale of Two Cities*

We have lived with the acquired immunodeficiency syndrome
(AIDS) epidemic, witnessing every day its paradoxes. People living
with the human immunodeficiency virus (HIV) not only live with the
fear, pain, and uncertainty of the disease, they also endure prejudice,
scorn, and rejection by society. Yet, persons living with HIV give support and encouragement to others and, by their example, change igno-
rance and prejudice to understanding and compassion. Our patients
have enriched our lives and redefined the limits of our professions.

An orphaned child, known to have HIV, is welcomed into an
extended or foster family. A homosexual man, unwelcomed and dis-
dained by his natural family, is offered profound love and support from
his community. A woman, alone, struggling, neglecting her own needs
for her child, crying for help, finally finds others who listen and care.

The nurse, the social worker, the doctor, the psychologist, the outreach worker, the counselor, the volunteer often have been the only
family for many living with HIV. These colleagues, including the members and the staff of this panel, have quietly and persistently struggled
to provide compassionate care to people and families living with HIV.

These many generous acts of kindness, courage, and commitment,
and the people behind them, have inspired and guided us throughout
this guideline process. We are honored to be among those striving
in these "worst of times" toward a future without HIV, a true "best
of times."

Contents

Appendix B. Drug Dosing Information

Appendix C

Index

Tables

Executive Summary

Introduction

The Agency for Health Care Policy and Research (AHCPR) convened a multidisciplinary, private-sector panel of physicians, dentists, nurses, nurse practitioners, physician assistants, social workers, and medical consumers to create a guideline for the evaluation and management of early human immunodeficiency virus (HIV) infection. The panel limited its focus to early HIV infection because (a) recognition of early infection is becoming more common; (b) the prevalence of early HIV infection is increasing in proportion to later stages of infection; (c) medical intervention in the early stage of HIV infection may be most effective in delaying life-threatening symptoms; and (d) early patient education often facilitates increased patient involvement in treatment and better access to services and helps prevent further spread of the disease.

This guideline contains panel recommendations, made as a result of an exhaustive search and analysis of relevant literature, clinical experience, peer review, public testimony, and a feasibility review. The guideline, which seeks to serve primary care providers as well as those with HIV infection, consists of five parts: *Clinical Practice Guideline,* which contains detailed recommendations and is primarily aimed at health care providers; *Guideline Report,* which contains supporting technical materials; *Quick Reference Guide for Clinicians,* a summary of the key components of the *Clinical Practice Guideline; HIV and Your Child,* a pamphlet that provides information for parents and guardians of infected children; and *Understanding HIV,* a pamphlet that provides information for adolescents and adults with HIV infection and their families and friends.

The guideline is not a comprehensive guide to early HIV care. Rather, it provides detailed recommendations for: (a) counseling related to disclosure of HIV status; (b) medical evaluation and management of early HIV infection and selected conditions in adults, adolescents, infants, and children; and (c) case management. The guideline also suggests strategies for addressing challenges in providing and accessing appropriate and comprehensive early HIV care. Because advances in the management of HIV infection are occurring at a rapid pace, providers should seek frequent updates.

Recommendations were based whenever possible on published evidence. Where evidence was inadequate to form the basis for a recommendation, the panel relied on expert opinion and consensus. Each recommendation is followed by a rating that indicates the extent to which it is evidence based. To complement the text, eight algorithms

1

(Appendix A) visually represent the selected aspects of evaluation and management of early HIV infection. The guideline also lists sources of further information and State reporting requirements.

Disclosure

Disclosure is defined in two ways: (a) provider disclosure of HIV status to the patient and, in the case of HIV-infected children, to parents or guardians; and, where mandatory or necessary, to health or other agencies; and (b) the patient's voluntary disclosure of his or her HIV status to individuals and agencies.

When HIV status is disclosed to the patient, counseling should include discussion of psychosocial and medical effects of HIV, available therapies, and support services. The patient should be informed of Federal, State, and local reporting requirements and of potential advantages and disadvantages of voluntary disclosure to family, friends, associates, and groups. Patients should be strongly encouraged to disclose their HIV status to significant others, particularly sex and needle-sharing partners, to prevent further transmission of HIV.

Assessments of the need for case management and mental health treatment including crisis management should be included in these initial counseling sessions. Ongoing counseling is required as an integral part of medical management.

Care of Adults and Adolescents

Essential components of early HIV care examined by this panel include: assessment of immune function; initiation of antiretroviral treatment and prophylaxis for *Pneumocystis carinii* pneumonia (PCP); evaluation and management of infection with *Mycobacterium tuberculosis* and syphilis; oral, eye, and gynecologic assessment; and reproductive counseling. Evaluation should begin with a medical, sexual, and substance use history, followed by a physical examination with attention to HIV-related complications. Providers caring for adolescents need to be cognizant of a range of age-specific issues, including assessment of physical maturity, psychosocial aspects of adolescence, and impediments to accessing care.

Immune status should be assessed by determining the number of CD4 cells. The number of CD4 cells should be measured every 6 months when the CD4 count is 600 cells/μl or above and at least every 3 months when the CD4 count is between 200 and 600 cells/μl. Antiretroviral therapy should be offered to all asymptomatic patients when the CD4 cell count falls below 500 cells/μl. PCP prophylaxis should be started when the CD4 count falls below 200 cells/μl, when there has been a prior episode of PCP, or in the presence of other specific signs or symptoms. Pregnant women with HIV infection should have CD4 cells measured at entry into prenatal care or at delivery if there is no prenatal care, and counts should be repeated every trimester if the count is between 200 and 600 cells/μl. Antiretroviral therapy should be offered when the CD4 count is less than 500 cells/μl, and PCP prophylaxis is recommended as for nonpregnant adults.

Patients should be screened for *M. tuberculosis* at the initial examination, irrespective of prior bacille Calmette-Guerin (BCG) vaccination. History of exposure to *M. tuberculosis* and prior tuberculosis (TB), including treatment, should be carefully ascertained. HIV-infected individuals should be screened for cutaneous anergy at the time of purified protein derivative (PPD) testing. Patients who are PPD-positive, are anergic, or have symptoms suggestive of TB should have a chest x-ray; if any abnormalities are noted on chest x-ray, followup should include sputum smears and cultures for mycobacteria. If the smear is positive for acid-fast organisms, the patient should be started on therapy immediately, taking into account local susceptibility patterns, and remain in therapy until definitive sputum culture results are known. Providers can foster treatment adherence by developing solid relationships with patients and by using directly observed therapy (DOT) or case management.

HIV-infected patients should be evaluated for syphilis as part of the initial assessment, starting with a careful history of syphilis and its treatment and with a nontreponemal test. In patients who have reactive nontreponemal tests, a treponemal test should be performed. Evaluation of cerebrospinal fluid (CSF) should be done whenever possible for patients with reactive treponemal serology. In HIV-infected individuals, treatment for all stages of syphilis except neurosyphilis should consist of three weekly doses of benzathine penicillin; patients with neurosyphilis should receive intravenous aqueous penicillin for 10 to 14 days. In HIV-infected pregnant women, assessment for syphilis should be performed at entry into prenatal care, during the third trimester, at delivery, or on exposure to or presentation with a sexually transmitted disease. Penicillin treatment should be completed at least 4 weeks before delivery to prevent congenital syphilis.

An oral examination should be conducted by the primary care provider at each visit; a dental examination by a dentist should be done at least two times per year.

An eye examination including a funduscopy should be conducted by the primary care provider at each office visit. Patients should be asked if they have experienced any visual disturbances and should be referred to a qualified eye doctor for any signs or symptoms suggestive of ocular cytomegalovirus infection (CMV).

Special Considerations for Treating Women

Clinical experience and available data suggest that care of HIV-infected women should include gynecologic evaluations, including a Papanicolaou (Pap) smear and rectovaginal examination, at least one time per year. Pregnant women should have a Pap smear at entry into prenatal care or as soon as possible after delivery. Patients with Pap smears that show atypical cells of undetermined significance, squamous intraepithelial lesions (SILs), and squamous carcinoma should be referred for colposcopy. Colposcopy should not be used as a screening tool in place of Pap smears.

Pregnancy counseling for HIV-infected women should be objective and nonjudgmental. Current data regarding perinatal transmission and the effects of pregnancy and childbirth on HIV progression should be included, as should a discussion of the potential long-term impact of pregnancy decisions on the family. Issues related to access of women to clinical trials and investigational treatments are discussed in the guideline, and strategies are offered for linking women to trials and investigational treatments when appropriate, given current barriers. The panel advises against breast-feeding by HIV-infected mothers in the United States.

Care of Infants and Children

HIV infection frequently progresses more rapidly in infants and children than in adults, and the disease characteristics are different. Early diagnosis and evaluation of the immune system are vital, and the disease must be managed aggressively.

HIV infection should be diagnosed early. HIV can be detected in the blood or body fluids of infants under 18 months of age with a viral culture, p24 antigen assay, or a polymerase chain reaction (PCR) assay. Infection in a child over 18 months of age can be determined with the enzyme-linked immunosorbent assay (ELISA) test and confirmed with the Western blot, as with adolescents and adults.

Immune status should be evaluated by a CD4 cell count and percentage at 1 month, at 3 months, and at 3-month intervals thereafter through 24 months of age. Older HIV-infected infants and children should have a CD4 count and percentage done as part of their initial evaluation for HIV infection and every 6 months thereafter. Prophylaxis for PCP is indicated after an episode of PCP or if the CD4 cell count or percentage falls below age-adjusted normal values. Antiretroviral therapy is indicated for all infants, children, and adolescents with symptomatic HIV infection or for any child with a CD4 count or percentage that falls below the age-adjusted values.

A neurologic assessment should be conducted at every visit. A baseline computerized axial tomography (CT) scan or magnetic resonance imaging (MRI) should be performed, where possible, in HIV-infected infants, children, and adolescents at the time of diagnosis of HIV infection. An age-related developmental assessment should be performed at initial assessment and repeated as recommended. Abnormal neurologic findings are an indication for repeated neuro-imaging study and a CSF evaluation. After exclusion of other diagnoses, infants and children with HIV-related central nervous system (CNS) disease should be treated with antiretroviral drugs.

Case Management

Efforts should be made to coordinate both medical care and support services for HIV-infected individuals either by the primary care provider or through a formal case-management system. In the early stages of HIV infection, many of the services required by patients will be community based; these services include assistance with housing and with occupational, legal, and financial matters. In the later stages of disease, the patient will require more medically oriented services. The primary care provider should develop contacts with existing case-management programs in the community and should participate in the case management of patients. Case-management programs should be administered by persons knowledgeable about both health services delivery and the clinical nature of HIV infection.

Access and Availability of HIV Care

Primary care providers and consumers should be aware of issues affecting access to and availability of care so that relevant barriers can be anticipated and overcome. The panel recommends a series of immediate short-term steps that may be taken on the societal level, as well as strategies for providers and patients which include:

- Become familiar with broad issues dealing with access to and availability of care, particularly with potential obstacles to obtaining care.

- Recognize and discuss specific obstacles that may arise given individual coverage parameters, including third-party and Medicaid limitations.

- Employ a case-management approach to care planning which includes development of care plans, linkage and advocacy services, and coordination of care.

- Participate in community- and organization-level incentive and recognition programs for providers of HIV care.

5

Overview

Introduction

The human immunodeficiency virus (HIV) epidemic, still young from a historical perspective, has already changed dramatically in the United States. Originally identified in homosexual men, it now increasingly affects men and women of all races, ethnicities, and sexual orientations, as well as infants, children, and adolescents. The obstacles to ensuring adequate care for these diverse populations, and the complexity of care for each individual, make HIV infection one of the greatest challenges of our time.

According to the World Health Organization (WHO, 1992), 30 to 40 million men, women, and children around the world will be infected with HIV by the year 2000. Others have estimated that this number could be as high as 110 million (Mann, Tarantola, and Netter, 1992). Infection with this virus begins a long process in which the immune system is gradually weakened and destroyed, leaving a person increasingly vulnerable to a range of infections that a normal immune system would successfully combat. By the turn of the century, acquired immunodeficiency syndrome (AIDS), which is the ultimate manifestation of infection with HIV, will be the third most common cause of death in the United States (WHO, 1992).

The toll exacted on the Nation by HIV and AIDS is enormous. In 1992, the care of patients with HIV infection cost the U.S. economy more than $10 billion in direct medical costs, time lost from work, and other indirect costs (Hellinger, 1992). In addition to the financial costs of HIV and AIDS, there are also great emotional and psychological pressures on individuals and families as they attempt to cope with this devastating disease and on society as it grapples with an epidemic that is spreading to an increasingly diverse population.

The focus for this guideline is the evaluation and management of selected aspects of early HIV infection. Our initial inclination was to make this guideline comprehensive. Given that the course of the infection follows a continuum, people enter care at different stages, and care within each stage is complex, we asked ourselves repeatedly how we could limit ourselves to only selected aspects of one stage of HIV infection. From a practical standpoint, however, it was necessary to limit the focus. In selecting early infection, we considered the following:

- Asymptomatic or early HIV infection is becoming increasingly recognized, due in large part to more widespread HIV testing and earlier diagnosis.

7

■ During early infection, individuals with HIV are better able to learn about the disease and the resources available to them. This is also an important time to consult with their providers in making decisions regarding evaluation and treatment.

■ Early medical and psychosocial intervention is most effective in delaying the onset of life-threatening symptoms and diseases and in maintaining the patient in good health.

■ At this stage, there is an opportunity to provide education on preventing transmission of the virus.

During a patient's asymptomatic period of potentially a decade or more, there are a series of medical, psychological, and social interventions that providers can implement which can improve the patients' quality of life. For HIV-infected individuals and their families, however, fear of stigmatization or discrimination and lack of access to services may delay initial assessment and early intervention.

For the purposes of this guideline, the panel has defined early HIV infection as the stage without major medical symptoms, although emotional or psychological difficulties are likely to be present. Within this definition of early infection, the panel identified numerous topics that needed intensive review, from which 14 were selected. Thus, the guideline is not comprehensive; rather, it provides detailed recommendations for selected aspects of early care.

This guideline is for both primary care providers and recipients of care. In the initial years of the epidemic, the most severe complications of HIV infection received the most attention. The focus has now evolved to emphasize outpatient care, health maintenance, prevention of hospitalization, and the integration of the patient and loved ones into a system that provides supportive services. Thus, primary care providers must be prepared to diagnose HIV infection, disclose test results, and evaluate and manage early infection.

In the guideline, the panel has emphasized that coordination of care is the responsibility of the primary care provider. Fragmentation of care is one of the most common problems faced by people living with HIV. The primary care provider must assume the responsibility for ensuring coordinated care. However, when multiple acute and chronic needs exist for a patient, the primary care provider may be assisted by a case management system. With these roles in mind, we defined "primary care provider" in the broadest sense: the person who assumes the major medical and coordinating role in the patient's care.

Through this guideline, the panel hopes to demystify HIV care. Early HIV infection does not require an array of practitioners. The primary care provider can and should develop the skills to assume this role. The panel recognizes potential difficulties: discomfort with discussion of personal behaviors including sexual practices and substance use, the challenge of acquiring new diagnostic and treatment skills, and the effort needed to remain current with a rapidly evolving field. To this end, this guideline can be considered a resource for providers.

Throughout the guideline, emphasis is placed on the provider and patient working together as a team to plan care. Although certain individuals may prefer that the provider make decisions and direct care, HIV-infected persons and their providers should share information about HIV infection and care options. This is particularly true in areas outside the direct purview of the provider, such as self-care (ensuring proper nutrition, sleep, and housing and living conditions) and risk reduction.

The panel has emphasized the importance of access to promising new drugs and therapies for the treatment of HIV infection. Patients have been clamoring for help in their struggle against this disease. Unfortunately, enrollment in clinical trials has been slow in reaching women, adolescents, minorities, and, in particular, people of color. Continued efforts are needed to remove the obstacles that hinder participation of these patients in trials, such as lack of support services, outreach, and education in existing programs. Linking clinical trials to the primary care setting is essential. Providers are responsible for sharing with their patients current information on these trials and treatments and facilitating access to them.

HIV infection has elements common to all patients and others specific to certain subpopulations. Likewise, there are evaluation and management processes and approaches unique to the special conditions, belief systems, and needs of each patient. For example, the evaluation and monitoring of CD4 cells is central to the management of HIV infection for all patients; however, CD4 testing for pregnant women and infants presents special issues. Routine oral and eye care is recommended for all patients, as is the monitoring of tuberculosis (TB) and syphilis. All women require gynecologic assessments and pregnancy counseling. For infants and children, special attention is necessary for identification and confirmation of HIV infection and for monitoring neurologic growth and development. Finally, adolescents share features common to all infected populations while experiencing their own unique challenges.

HIV affects the whole family, whether one or all of its members are HIV infected. Crises occur on a regular basis: the hospitalization of a child, the loss of a parent or sibling, the accumulated toll of lacking needed services, the time and energy spent in seeking care, the orphaned child who needs a home.

Our central concerns must be to halt the epidemic and provide adequate care for those already affected. Those who are infected with

HIV still feel the pain of stigmatization and discrimination while suffering from lack of access to care. Our priorities must include:

- Developing sound and innovative public health programs to prevent further transmission of the virus, such as needle-exchange programs and school-based education regarding HIV and its transmission.

- Providing resources adequate to allow comprehensive and compassionate care.

- Calling for an end to discrimination against, and stigmatization of, those at risk for and those with HIV infection, including an end to travel restrictions.

- Promoting the development of a generation of informed citizens and providers interested in and committed to treating this disease, who are cognizant of but do not exaggerate the risk of transmission.

- Assuring funding that matches the gravity of this epidemic.

Organization of the Guideline

The guideline is organized into six major sections. The first includes disclosure of HIV status, an issue that affects all persons living with HIV throughout the course of their disease. The second discusses general management of the adult patient. The third discusses care for adolescents. The fourth focuses on infants and children. The fifth includes recommendations for use in case management for persons living with HIV. The last section concerns access to health care for persons with HIV. Clearly, we as a society must pursue approaches that aim to remove barriers to accessing early HIV care. On the individual level, the panel believes that by recognizing and understanding barriers to obtaining early HIV care, providers and consumers can employ strategies to maximize access to care and utilize to the fullest the care that is available.

Guideline Development Methodology

The guideline is the product of an intensive 20-month effort. During this time, the panel held two public forums and five panel meetings and produced six drafts of the guideline. The guideline development process included selection of panel co-chairs and panelists, identification of the topics to be addressed in the guideline, a comprehensive search and review of the published literature, public forums, external peer review of the guideline, and pilot review of documents associated with the guideline (e.g., *Understanding HIV* and *HIV and*

Your Child, the consumer versions of the guideline; and the *Quick Reference Guide for Clinicians).*

Co-chairs Wafaa El-Sadr, MD, MPH, and James M. Oleske, MD, MPH, were appointed by the Administrator, Agency for Health Care Policy and Research (AHCPR). Panelists were nominated in response to an announcement in the *Federal Register.* Significant experience with HIV infection and expertise in a discipline relevant to HIV care was a prerequisite for panel membership.

Selecting Topics for Inclusion in the Guideline_____

At its first meeting, the panel agreed to focus on the evaluation and management of early HIV infection. Two factors were important in determining the scope of the guideline within this broader area. First, because of the urgent need for clinical guidelines for HIV-related care, the panel had to develop the guideline relatively quickly (approximately 1 year). Second, AHCPR was committed to a rigorous approach to guideline development, including an exhaustive review of the pertinent literature. These constraints precluded the development of recommendations that included all aspects of the evaluation and management of early HIV infection, and the panel thus limited its focus to a subset of topics.

The panel employed a five-step process to identify the topics to include in the guideline. First, panelists compiled a master list of relevant topics. The co-chairs then organized this master list into four categories and separated the panelists into four corresponding subpanels: (1) issues relating to adults with HIV infection; (2) issues pertaining to children and adolescents with HIV infection; (3) special concerns relevant to women with HIV infection; and (4) broad HIV-related issues concerning knowledge, attitudes, and practices.

The subpanelists were asked to score each topic in their subpanel area according to six attributes: (1) importance of the issue according to the consumer, (2) severity of the problem in clinical terms, (3) universality of the problem across geographic areas and subpopulations, (4) uncertainty in practice, (5) feasibility of changing provider behavior, and (6) feasibility of mobilizing societal resources necessary for changes. These six attributes were designed to reflect the factors believed to be important in developing guidelines that lead to improved outcomes (Institute of Medicine, 1990). In addition, the methodologists rated each topic in terms of the technical feasibility of addressing it with structured analytic approaches such as decision analysis or meta-analysis. Finally, the sum of the seven scores for each topic were scaled and used to rank each topic. Fourteen areas were selected to be the basis of the guideline.

Searching and Reviewing the Literature_____

The 14 selected topics were submitted to the National Library of Medicine (NLM) for a literature search. The co-chairs, in consultation with their staffs and NLM personnel, selected inclusion and exclusion search criteria. The search terms used by the library are available in a technical report. In addition, for selected questions that were judged to be particularly complex, the linkage between the intervention and the health outcomes of interest were identified explicitly using formal methods for structuring problems (Owens and Nease, 1993).

The library search identified nearly 36,000 abstracts from 1981 through 1992. A first review of all the abstracts was made by the co-chairs and research staff to identify and exclude those citations not relevant to the guideline topics; relevant abstracts were retained for further review. This review reduced the number of citations to 2,831. A second review excluded additional citations not relevant to the guideline. Additional citations through August 1993 were also reviewed. All articles were subjected to the same review process, described below, regardless of the method by which they were identified.

The selected articles were reviewed for both clinical content and methodologic quality. The clinical content review was done by at least one member of the panel; the reviews for methodologic quality were performed by consultants with training in epidemiology. Reviews were returned to the co-chairs and collated by the research staff. A computerized data base was developed which included selected items from the two reviews. Summary tables for each topic were prepared for use by the panel.

Developing Recommendations_____

The panelists used published data to the greatest extent possible when formulating recommendations. Expert opinion was used as a basis for recommendations only when published studies did not address the topic sufficiently or did not provide definitive evidence. In some cases, the panelists chose not to make recommendations because of insufficient evidence and no consensus among experts. Each recommendation was rated and labeled according to the degree to which it was data based:

- Supported by evidence: Evidence from at least one well- designed published randomized controlled trial in the population for which the recommendation is made; or, for recommendations to provide information, results from at least one well-designed published population-based study.

■ Suggested by evidence: Consistent results from other study designs or studies in populations other than that for which the recommendation is made.

■ Expert opinion: Expert clinical experience described in the literature or derived from consensus of panel members.

In addition to the clinical recommendations addressed in the guideline, the panel elected to analyze three areas it deemed crucial to the appropriate management of persons with early HIV infection: access and availability of services, adherence to TB treatment regimens, and inclusion of women in HIV-related clinical trials. These statements were developed by the panel in consultation with a health policy analyst.

Eliciting and Addressing Public Opinion

Before the second panel meeting, two open forums, one in San Francisco and one in New York City, were held to receive input from the general public. A variety of concerns were raised by providers from many disciplines including physicians, public health workers, nurses, dietitians, and psychotherapists; activist groups; individual medical consumers; and other concerned parties. Suggestions from the two public forums were incorporated into the guideline, when appropriate.

External Review of the Guideline

The third draft of the guideline was circulated to 45 outside peer reviewers nominated by the panelists and by AHCPR. Peer reviewers included clinicians, AIDS program directors, social workers, counselors, health educators, researchers with clinical experience, consumers, and key personnel at selected Federal agencies (Centers for Disease Control and Prevention, Health Resources and Services Administration, National Institutes of Health, Food and Drug Administration, President's Transitional Team). Reviewers were asked to assess the guideline based on five criteria: validity, reliability, clarity, clinical applicability, and utility. The reviewers were encouraged to provide additional comments. The co-chairs synthesized the responses and, in consultation with appropriate panelists, incorporated selected comments of the peer reviewers.

In addition to the peer review of the guideline, 25 consumers and 16 providers performed a feasibility review of the consumer brochures and the quick reference guide for clinicians. As a followup to this review, about 100 HIV-positive men and women and parents and guardians of HIV-positive children participated in focus groups to evaluate the consumer guides. Comments obtained during the preliminary review and the focus groups were used to enhance the appropriateness and usefulness of these documents.

1 Guideline: Disclosure of HIV Status

Introduction

The disclosure of human immunodeficiency virus (HIV) test results is a critical event in the provider/patient relationship. This event represents the first knowledge of HIV status for the patient and also initiates an ongoing, long-term relationship between provider and patient. This relationship ultimately will be shaped by the actual and anticipated HIV-related needs of the patient (Goldschmidt and Legg, 1991).

In this guideline, the phrase "disclosure counseling" is used to apply to the interactions that arise as part of communicating an individual's HIV status. These interactions include:

- The provider informing the patient of HIV test results for the first time and providing appropriate counseling (post-test counseling).

- The provider reporting a patient's HIV results to government and service agencies.

- The patient revealing HIV status to a partner (partner notification), friends and family, employers, and private and public agencies, such as health insurance companies and government entitlement programs.

- Parents or guardians telling an infected child and others in the family about the child's infection.

Disclosure counseling concerning HIV test results, by providers to patients and by patients to others, sets the tone and foundation for patients' acceptance, knowledge base, and attitudes about their own HIV infection. This foundation in turn may dramatically affect patients' quality of life and their ability to care for themselves. In this section, recommendations for disclosure of HIV status are presented. We believe that these recommendations apply to all persons affected by HIV infection regardless of age, ethnicity, sex, or socioeconomic status, including patients, families, guardians, significant others, and caregivers.

Utilization of these recommendations begins after appropriate pretest counseling and informed consent have been made available to the patient. Specific issues relating to people with a negative HIV test result, disclosure of HIV status by health care workers, and disclosure of HIV status in day care and school settings need to be examined by subsequent panels.

15

We have separated disclosure counseling into three categories. In the first category, the provider discloses to the patient and, when appropriate, to partners, government, or service agencies. In the second category, the patient discloses to others, including public and private regulatory and service agencies. It should be noted that sometimes a patient discloses to a provider. This may happen when the patient has been tested in one location and seeks care in another. Although this situation is not discussed explicitly in this guideline, the considerations of the provider are the same as those described for other provider-patient interactions. In the third category, we discuss the provider's role in assisting parents or guardians in decisionmaking regarding disclosure of a child's or adolescent's HIV status to the child or adolescent and to other family members.

In the discussion that follows, disclosure counseling is assumed to be an ongoing process that is in the hands of a single provider. In reality, the initial provider may or may not maintain this role throughout the disclosure process. Users, therefore, will need to tailor the recommendations to fit their individual circumstances.

Disclosure Counseling by Providers

Disclosure to Patients

Recommendation: In planning the disclosure of the patient's HIV status to a patient or parent/guardian, the primary care provider should assess the degree to which the patient or parent/guardian is prepared to receive the results. If necessary, the content of pretest counseling and the process by which informed consent was obtained should be reviewed. The provider should discuss with the patient or parent/ guardian the natural history of HIV infection, the potential effects of HIV infection on physical and mental health, the role of health maintenance, and the availability of treatments. An assessment should be made of the patient's social, demographic, cultural, and psychological characteristics, which may relate to coping with a positive HIV antibody test. The provider may conduct these discussions or may seek the assistance of an individual with HIV counseling experience. For adolescent minors, the presence of a supportive adult during disclosure counseling is advantageous and should be encouraged. Disclosure counseling should occur face-to-face. (Suggested by evidence)

The published literature on counseling shows that, in general, patients are better able to cope with test results if they are prepared and informed by pretest counseling (Brown, Barton, Cutland et al., 1990; Futterman and Hein, 1990). The panel extrapolates from this general case to HIV infection: that disclosure of HIV test results to a patient for the first time will be considerably easier if the individual already understands the basic facts about HIV infection and HIV testing. Although this information should have been imparted during pretest counseling, the provider should use the first part of the disclosure counseling session to ascertain the level of understanding on the part of the patient and ensure full understanding. In addition, when disclosing an infant's HIV status to the parents or guardian, the provider needs to be aware that this information may be the initial recognition of HIV infection in the mother and possibly other members of the family.

Multiple additional factors affect a patient's ability to cope with HIV test results. These factors include age, sex, physical and mental health status, sexual orientation, availability of support systems, acknowledgment of prior exposure to HIV, perception of partner acceptance, beliefs and preferences with regard to religion and health care, circumstances under which HIV testing is performed (mandatory vs. voluntary), and the setting in which the information is shared (Brown, Barton, Cutland et al., 1990; Jones, Wykoff, Hollis et al., 1990; O'Dell, 1988; Pazen, 1991; Rekart, Knowles, Spencer, and Pengelly, 1990). The patient's status with regard to these factors will affect the future course of health care, subsequent counseling and disclosure, and the ability of the patient to care for him/herself and change his or her behavior. Thus, although certain elements of the discussion will be common across patients (e.g., the prevention of transmission), the provider should also tailor the content of posttest counseling to meet individual needs. Discussions with women, for example, should include potential gynecologic and obstetric complications of HIV infection. Housing issues will need to be addressed with poor or disenfranchised patients; and for children and adolescents, age-specific issues related to disclosure, including whether testing was voluntary or mandatory, need to be considered (AIDS and Adolescents' Network of New York, 1992; Futterman and Hein, 1990; Hein and Futterman, 1991; Kipke, Futterman, and Hein, 1990). (See also Caring for Adolescents with Early HIV Infection, Chapter 3.)

Recommendation: The disclosure counseling process is an opportunity to provide immediate interventions and involve the patient in ongoing medical, mental health, social, and family support networks. Immediate interventions should include assessing patients for the potential for violence to themselves or others; ensuring that patients receive a thorough evaluation, staging, and initial care; informing the patient of ongoing availability of services; scheduling the next appointment; addressing prevention of further HIV transmission; assessing the availability of an immediate support person (lover, partner, significant other, roommate, child, friend, parent, spouse,

spiritual support person) and other care providers; and providing available local and national sources of information. The provider should make appropriate referrals for any ongoing services that cannot be obtained on site. (Expert opinion)

Existing evidence documents that reactions to discussion of HIV status are highly individual and unpredictable; thus, the provider should be equipped to secure short-term support for the patient. Specifically, studies indicate that knowledge of HIV status may result in behaviors such as increased suicidal ideation or attempts, drug use, and unsafe sexual activity (Coates and Lo, 1990; Elmslie, Shearman, and Busing, 1989; Fortin, Boyer, Duval et al., 1990; Magallon, 1987). In the panel's experience, however, there may also be an increase in positive behaviors, such as enrollment into drug treatment programs and adoption of safer sexual and drug-injecting practices.

Irrespective of the patient's reaction, the provider should recognize that disclosure counseling can be viewed as a point of entry into the HIV-related health care and social support system, and this contact should be used to its maximum potential in terms of introducing the patient to services and systems. Resource telephone numbers are listed in Appendix C-1.

Provider Disclosure to Agencies_____

Recommendation: Primary care providers should be aware of Federal, State, and local HIV reporting requirements, educate their patients about them, and ensure that patients are aware of the extent and the limits of HIV test result confidentiality. (Expert opinion)

At this time, all States and the District of Columbia require reporting of patients meeting the Centers for Disease Control and Prevention (CDC) surveillance case definition of AIDS (CDC, 1992a). Appendix C-2 lists the current HIV infection reporting requirements for all States.

Providers are responsible for providing their patients with information on their State's mandatory or voluntary HIV reporting requirements. Even in States without mandatory reporting of HIV status, the provider should inform the patient that once a diagnosis of AIDS is determined, the patient must be reported to the State health department. Such individuals must also be reported anonymously to the CDC (CDC, 1992a). Further, both TB and syphilis, which may occur in HIV-infected patients, are reportable in all jurisdictions, and such reporting will trigger disclosure of limited information to a health department.

The provider should develop recordkeeping systems appropriate for maintaining the patient's confidentiality and discuss any limitations with their patient. The patient should be made aware that upon death, AIDS may be entered as a cause of death on the death certificate and that family members and others may thus become aware of the diagnosis. Finally, the provider should remain acutely conscious of the potential discrimination that sometimes occurs through inadvertent disclosure.

Published information on the legal implications of disclosure of HIV infection focuses on the ethical balance between patient confidentiality and the "duty to warn" (Brennan, 1989; Casswell, 1989; Melroe, 1990; Reamer, 1991). The "duty to warn" involves the obligation to disclose a patient's status by a provider or agency to others potentially at risk of infection. Whereas State law may require mandatory reporting of HIV status or AIDS diagnosis to public health agencies, there are no legal requirements for providers or agencies to further inform partners or others at risk (Bayer and Toomey, 1992). Although providers have to weigh the ethical imperatives and legal requirements, case law relating this dilemma specifically to the HIV epidemic is still limited.

Disclosure by Patients to Other Individuals and Agencies

Recommendation: Primary care providers should assist patients in understanding the advantages and disadvantages of disclosing their HIV status to others by providing counseling, including factual information, opportunities for patient education and dialog, and referrals as needed. Patients should be informed of the potential for discriminatory practices against persons with HIV. (Expert opinion)

Primary care providers can help their patients appreciate why disclosure and discussion of their HIV infection may be useful in some situations and potentially detrimental in others. In some States, disclosure of HIV infection will permit enhanced entitlement benefits (Bayer and Toomey, 1992). Disclosure to significant others (in the case of adolescents, to supportive parents, guardians, or other adults) may result in increased social support or in allowing a significant other to decide whether to seek HIV testing. Conversely, disclosure may result in housing discrimination, loss of employment, loss of child custody, reduction or cessation of health benefits, or rejection by a potential employer or significant other (Feldsman, Tucker, Leifer et al., 1992; Hein and Futterman, 1991; Lo, Steinbrook, Cooke et al., 1989; Tasker, 1992).

Recommendation: Patients should be strongly advised and encouraged to disclose their HIV status to significant others, particularly sexual and needle-sharing partners. Providers may assist in this process if desired by patients, either directly or through referral to State or municipal partner-notification programs, if available. (Suggested by evidence)

Disclosure of HIV infection to significant others is often important to allow others at risk to be counseled and tested, obtain early intervention, and prevent further transmission of the virus. Studies have shown that although patients may prefer to inform partners of their HIV infection themselves, more partners are notified if a health care worker initiates the contact (Jones, Wykoff, Hollis et al., 1990). A review of partner-notification systems across the United States and parts of Europe indicated that there are ongoing evaluations of different approaches to partner notification (Toomey and Cates, 1989). The results of these studies may shed additional light on the effectiveness of different notification systems; however, ultimately, such results must be interpreted and applied in the context of local attitudes and practices relative to patient confidentiality. It should be noted here that partner-notification systems universally require personnel over and above the primary care provider.

It is important for the provider to be aware of the potential for domestic violence within intimate relationships where one or both partners are infected by HIV (Worth, 1989). Although there is concern regarding HIV infection and domestic violence, there is a body of literature regarding violence associated with substance use and violence directed toward women by spouse, partner, or other family member (Karan, 1989). Domestic violence may occur in all types of relationships: heterosexual, homosexual, and parent-child. The potential for violence highlights the need for skilled and sensitive assessment by the provider (House Select Committee, 1992; Novello and Allen, 1991). The National Association of People with AIDS and the National Gay and Lesbian Task Force are two organizations currently collecting data regarding violence associated with HIV infection.

Disclosure of Child's HIV Status by Parent or Guardian

Recommendation: The provider should assist parents and guardians in making decisions regarding disclosure of HIV infection to the infected child or adolescent and other family members. This assistance should consist of educating parents and guardians and working together with them to assure that needed support services are available and in place during the process of disclosure. (Expert opinion)

Disclosure of HIV diagnosis to an infected child is a difficult task for parents and guardians. Many factors, most of which have not been rigorously examined, enter into this process. When a child is very young or in the asymptomatic stage of the infection, disclosure may not be necessary. As the child becomes older or more symptomatic, it becomes more difficult as well as inadvisable to withhold discussion of diagnosis with the child. By early adolescence, HIV-infected youths should be informed of their status. After the HIV diagnosis is disclosed to a child or adolescent, problems may arise including subsequent inadvertent disclosure to others. In addition, the child or adolescent, like an adult, may become depressed or withdrawn as a result of this knowledge (Lipson, 1993).

Disclosure to infected children is an ongoing process which usually begins at around the age of 5. This may vary, however, depending on the child's developmental stage. Often, additional support services are needed by the child and the family to cope with this information. The provider can be effective in assisting the family to secure these services in anticipation of disclosure (Boland, Tasker, Evans, and Keresztes, 1987; Burr and Emery, in press; National Pediatric HIV Resource Center, 1992; Tasker, 1992).

Areas for Future Research

The panel identified the following research topics in the area of disclosure counseling:

- Assessment of counseling methodology.

- Evaluation of partner notification programs.

- Systematic assessment of issues in disclosure to children and adolescents.

2 Guideline: Early HIV Infection in Adults

Introduction

This chapter deals with the medical evaluation and management of adults[1] with HIV infection and is predicated on the hope that the provider and consumer will identify HIV infection early. Early identification provides an opportunity for an overall medical and psychological assessment to define the immediate and long-term needs of HIV-infected individuals and thereby maximize the length and quality of life.

In the evaluation and management of individuals with early HIV infection, the panel believes that in addition to assessing immune function (e.g., CD4 cell testing) and initiating antiretroviral treatment and *Pneumocystis carinii* pneumonia (PCP) prophylaxis, many other concerns are of central importance. These include the detection and treatment of other infections (e.g., tuberculosis [TB] and syphilis), oral care, eye care, the provision of preventive measures including immunizations, the evaluation and management of the patient's psychological and social needs, and the prevention of further transmission of HIV infection.

Detailed medical history-taking is crucial and should emphasize review of HIV test result, previous infections (including opportunistic infections [OIs]), and sexual and substance use history. A comprehensive physical examination—including attention to eye and oral examination, neurologic examination, and careful skin and lymph node assessment, as well as HIV-associated signs and symptoms (such as weight loss)—allow the provider to define the stage of HIV infection and determine the appropriate course of management and treatment for the individual patient. These steps, when accompanied by a discussion focusing on the concerns and fears of the patient (such as risk of transmission of infection to others, insurance coverage, and questions regarding prognosis), create an opportunity to provide HIV-infected individuals with information regarding the course of the infection, new treatments, anticipated symptoms and signs, and available community resources. In this context, the provider and the patient can work together as partners to develop a future care plan that prepares both for anticipated events and changes based on medical advances and new discoveries.

---

[1]Throughout this section and associated algorithms, the term "adult" includes infected adolescents who are Tanner stage IV or V; see Chapter 3: Caring for Adolescents with HIV Infection.

This chapter provides detailed recommendations for selected aspects of early HIV care for adults. It must be noted that these selected aspects do not represent a comprehensive overview of early HIV care. This guideline addresses items that must be included in all evaluations; it does not address others which also need attention. Algorithm 1 (Appendix A), depicts the selected aspects of evaluating and managing adults with early HIV infection which are covered in this guideline.

Topics discussed in this chapter include: the uses and timing of CD4 testing (for monitoring disease progression and initiation of specific therapies), evaluation and management of infection with TB and syphilis, and oral and eye examinations. This section also provides a discussion of management issues unique to women with HIV, such as the use and timing of Papanicolaou (Pap) smears and the role of reproductive and pregnancy counseling. In addition, several issues relevant to HIV-infected pregnant women, including CD4 testing, evaluation and management of syphilis, and enrollment into clinical drug trials, are discussed.

Many additional clinical assessments and laboratory examinations are an integral part of the evaluation and management of early HIV infection. Many of these issues were not reviewed by the panel but should be incorporated into every early HIV care plan. Future panels may address these important issues.

Areas for Future Research

The panel identified the following issues for future research:

- Study of indicators for changing antiretroviral agents.

- Prospective study of management of syphilis in HIV-infected individuals.

- Evaluation of the natural history and treatment of cervical (Pap smear) abnormalities in HIV-infected women.

- Evaluation of various models of engaging women and injection drug users in treatment programs and clinical trials.

- Studies of the impact of various treatments on the quality of life of patients.

Monitoring CD4 Lymphocytes and Initiating Antiretroviral Therapy and PCP Prophylaxis

The assessment of immune status by measuring CD4 lymphocyte count is important for establishing the stage of HIV infection and prognosis of disease and determining the appropriateness of initiating both antiretroviral therapy and prophylaxis for PCP and other OIs. The framework for this is discussed below and presented in Algorithm 2 (Appendix A). Special information on CD4 testing and treatment for pregnant women with HIV infection is provided at the end of this section and in Algorithm 3 (Appendix A). It is crucial that the provider become acquainted with newly recognized treatment options as they become available and provide patients with access to promising and appropriate ones. Decisions to initiate therapy should follow a discussion with the patient of available data and options. Drugs and doses described in this chapter are detailed in Appendix B.

Laboratory Evaluation of Immune Function_____

Recommendation: An HIV-infected individual should have an assessment of immune status as part of a complete initial evaluation. Measurement of the number of CD4 lymphocytes should be the primary test for monitoring immune function. Measurement of the number of CD4 cells should be done once every 6 months when the CD4 count is greater than 600 cells/μl and at least every 3 months when the CD4 count is between 200 and 600 cells/μl. Obtaining CD4 counts may be desirable at more frequent intervals if there is evidence of rapid decline or with increasing symptoms. Ongoing monitoring of CD4 counts below 200 cells/μl at least every 3 months may be necessary to monitor the effect of antiretroviral therapy and for initiation of new preventive and therapeutic strategies. (Expert opinion)

CD4 lymphocyte measurement is useful for determining stage of illness, risk of progression, and timing for the initiation of both antiretroviral therapy and prophylaxis for PCP and other OIs. Measurement of immune function is also used in determining eligibility for clinical trials and as part of the determination of disability status. Currently, CD4 counts for mature adolescents are assumed to be similar to adults (see Chapter 3, Caring for Adolescents with Early HIV Infection).

Although knowledge of both percentage and number of CD4 lymphocytes may be useful in monitoring the immune system, the preponderance of literature supports the use of CD4 counts (Stein, Korvick, and Vermund, 1992). Significant variation in CD4 lymphocyte measurements does occur regardless of whether the number or percentage of CD4 lymphocytes is used as the standard of measurement. The Multicenter AIDS Cohort Study (MACS) established a quality control program for measurement of CD4 lymphocytes and found variations within centers, between centers, and in the same patients (Kaslow, 1987). To keep variability to a minimum, laboratories should adhere to rigorous quality control programs (CDC, 1992b).

Although there are indications that monitoring the percentage of CD4 cells is less subject to variability than monitoring the number of CD4 cells (Kaslow, 1987; Parker, 1988), the CD4 count has been the criterion widely used to correlate with clinical effectiveness in clinical studies. In addition, published guidelines on the use of antiretroviral therapies and PCP prophylaxis and other preventive therapies in adults are based on CD4 counts, not percentages. We therefore recommend measurement of the number of CD4 lymphocytes in individuals with HIV infection as the routine test for monitoring immune status. The value of this test will be improved when it is better standardized, and research efforts in this area should be supported, including the identification of other surrogate markers of immune function.

The panel discourages CD4 lymphocyte testing more frequently than is necessary for clinical decisionmaking. Consistent with the guidelines promulgated by the National Institute of Allergy and Infectious Diseases (NIAID), the panel recommends testing once every 6 months when CD4 counts are > 600 cells/μl (National Institutes of Health [NIH], 1990). However, when an individual has shown great variability in test results or when a patient is close to a point when a clinical intervention may be indicated, the panel recommends testing at least every 3 months.

Ongoing single, combination, and sequential antiretroviral clinical trials that monitor the rate of decline in CD4 counts and percentages may provide additional information about the use of CD4 counts in monitoring progression of disease. More research is needed to determine the clinical impact of these changes in CD4 cells.

A number of studies suggest that other tests may be valuable in monitoring progression of HIV infection. These include p24 antigen, beta-2-microglobulin, neopterin, and CD8 cell measurement (Fahey, Taylor, Detels et al., 1990; MacDonell, Chmiel, Poggensee et al., 1990; Polk, 1987). At this time, available information does not support their routine use in the evaluation of the newly diagnosed HIV-infected individual. However, they may play an adjunctive role in clinical decisionmaking and evaluation of progression of disease.

Using CD4 Cell Count to Time Initiation of Antiretroviral Therapy

Recommendation: Antiretroviral therapy should be deferred for asymptomatic individuals with early HIV infection and CD4 counts greater than 500 cells/μl. Antiretroviral therapy with zidovudine should be offered to all asymptomatic HIV-infected individuals with CD4 counts less than 500 cells/μl. (Suggested by evidence)

Recommendation: Decisions regarding immediate initiation or deferral of treatment should be made jointly by the provider and patient following a discussion of risks and benefits. (Expert opinion)

In 1987, antiretroviral therapy with the nucleoside analog zidovudine (3'-azido-3'-deoxythymidine, formerly azidothymidine [AZT], now ZDV) was found to be effective in delaying the onset of OIs and prolonging survival in patients with AIDS and advanced HIV disease (Fischl, Richman, and Grieco, 1987). In 1990, the benefit of ZDV in individuals who were asymptomatic with CD4 lymphocyte counts less than 500 cells/ml was demonstrated (Volberding, Lagakos, Koch et al., 1990). Although the latter study demonstrated a significant delay in progression to AIDS or advanced HIV disease, the study did not demonstrate a difference in mortality within 2 years with use of ZDV. Further followup of these patients is ongoing. This study also showed that the group treated with the lower dose of ZDV (500 mg per day) experienced significantly less toxicity than the group treated with the higher dose. As a result of this finding, 500-600 mg per day of ZDV is the recommended dose for both symptomatic and asymptomatic individuals with CD4 counts less than 500 cells/ml.[2] As a part of this recommendation, it was suggested that the stability of the CD4 count be ensured by promptly repeating the count prior to the initiation of therapy (NIH, 1990).

A Veterans Administration-sponsored randomized trial of early vs. late treatment with ZDV (at doses of 1500 mg per day) in persons with mild, symptomatic HIV infection and CD4 counts between 200 and 500 cells/ml also showed delayed progression to AIDS, particularly for those with CD4 counts <300 cells/ml (Hamilton, Hartigan, Simberkoff et al., 1992). This latter study also did not demonstrate a survival benefit from early therapy.

Retrospective studies, however, support the beneficial effects of ZDV on survival of patients. Analysis of the MACS data suggests that early initiation of ZDV may prolong survival (Graham, Zeger, Park et al., 1992). This study analyzed data from 2,568 HIV-infected participants followed for 24 months. Mortality was significantly reduced in patients who received ZDV before the development of an AIDS diagnosis. This effect was in addition to the beneficial effect of prophylaxis for PCP. In addition, other retrospective studies confirmed the previous finding and also demonstrated a survival advantage with early

---

[2]Information included in this guideline may not represent Food and Drug Administration (FDA) approval or approved labeling for the particular products or indications in question. Specifically, the terms "safe" and "effective" may not be synonymous with the FDA-defined legal standards for product approval.

ZDV use in all racial groups (Merigan, Amato, and Balsley, 1991; Moore, Hidalgo, Sugland, and Chaisson, 1991; Moore, Keruly, Richman et al., 1992).

Preliminary results of the Concorde trial were recently published (Aboulker and Swart, 1993). In this study, 1,749 asymptomatic HIV-infected individuals were recruited and assigned randomly to groups receiving 1 g ZDV per day or to groups receiving a matching placebo. The CD4 count in individuals receiving ZDV rose to significantly higher levels than in those receiving a placebo. Although this study showed a beneficial effect of ZDV in delaying progression of disease at 1 year followup, there was no significant difference in clinical progression of HIV disease or in survival at 3-years followup.

Further studies are needed to determine the role of ZDV in asymptomatic HIV-infected individuals with CD4 counts >500 cells/μl. The Concorde study included a large number of asymptomatic patients with CD4 counts >500 cells/μl and did not demonstrate a beneficial effect of ZDV in terms of progression of disease or survival (Aboulker and Swart, 1993). A recently published study of asymptomatic individuals with CD4 cell counts >400 cells/μl (the Australian/European Study) suggested that ZDV was beneficial in prevention of minor symptoms of HIV and delay in drop of CD4 cells to <350 cells/μl (Cooper, Gatell, Kroon et al., 1993). However, the latter study did not demonstrate a benefit of ZDV in delay of progression to AIDS or severe HIV symptoms and did not report survival data.

At this time, the panel supports offering ZDV to individuals with CD4 counts <500 cells/μl. Nevertheless, it is essential that this decision be made in conjunction with the patient, who has been informed of the differing results across studies in terms of the effect of early treatment on progression of disease. Other issues to be considered in the decision to begin antiretroviral therapy in patients with early HIV infection include:

■ The results of published randomized studies, which have not shown that early treatment clearly influences survival.

■ The potential for reduction in OIs and hospitalizations as demonstrated in some studies.

■ The results of nonrandomized studies, which demonstrate beneficial effects on survival.

■ Potential changes in quality of life caused by the need to take multiple doses of medication.

■ Potential adverse drug effects.

■ Potential development of antiretroviral drug resistance.

■ The expanding availability of antiretroviral therapy (see recommendations below) which may provide future options for patients who choose immediate therapy.

■ The cost of medications.

■ The potential impact of initiating therapy on confidentiality.

It should be noted that for patients who decline antiretroviral therapy, close monitoring should be continued.

Recommendation: HIV-infected individuals who do not tolerate ZDV should be offered therapy with didanosine (ddI) or dideoxycitidine (ddC). Individuals who demonstrate progression of disease while receiving ZDV should be offered monotherapy with either ddI or ddC or combination therapy of ZDV with either ddI or ddC (see recommendation below). (Suggested by evidence)

Availability of other antiretroviral agents has provided alternatives to patients who are intolerant to ZDV or have not demonstrated favorable clinical or immunologic response to it. Although reasons for a lack of response to ZDV may be complex, it appears that resistance to ZDV may develop over time (Mayers, McCutchan, Sanders-Buell et al., 1992; Richman, 1990). Viral isolates from those in the earlier stages of HIV infection with higher CD4 counts developed reduced susceptibility to ZDV at slower rates than did isolates from people with AIDS or advanced disease. These observations of *in vitro* resistance have not been clearly correlated with clinical sequelae. Clinicians have used evidence of clinical deterioration, a decline in CD4 counts, or changes in other surrogate markers to decide when to change antiretroviral agents, despite a lack of definitive data to guide these decisions.

Intolerance to ZDV has been evaluated in clinical trials and includes anemia, neutropenia, nausea, insomnia, neuropathy, myopathy, liver dysfunction, headaches, and fatigue (see Appendix B-2). If anemia is significant, it can be managed by lowering the prescribed dose (a minimum of 300 mg per day), use of erythropoietin, or transfusion (Fischl, Galpin, Levine et al., 1990). Similarly, neutropenia can be managed by dose modification or potentially by use of colony-stimulating factors (Groopman, Mitsuyasu, DeLeo et al., 1989). Other adverse symptoms often diminish over time but, if persistent and severe, may necessitate dose modification or discontinuation of ZDV therapy (Kahn, Lagakos, Richman et al., 1992).

Recent data have provided several options to patients with intolerance or failure to respond to ZDV. ddI and ddC (or zalcitabine) are available options for individuals who do not tolerate ZDV or have failed to respond to it. Their toxicity profile is different from that of

ZDV; their major adverse effects are peripheral neuropathy, oral ulcerations (ddC), and pancreatitis, which can be fatal and is especially problematic in patients with preexisting pancreatitis or those who use excessive alcohol (ddI) (Cooley, Kunches, Saunders et al., 1990). Data have suggested that ddC may be slightly more effective than ddI in patients with advanced disease who are intolerant or have clinical progression while on ZDV (NIAID, 1993a).

Recommendation: HIV-infected individuals who are receiving and tolerating ZDV may benefit from a change of antiretroviral therapy to ddI. Combination therapy of ZDV with either ddI or ddC may provide another option. These therapeutic options should be discussed with and offered to patients. (Expert opinion)

A controversial issue is whether and when to change antiretroviral agents in patients who are doing well on ZDV. In a recent study, HIV-infected individuals who were asymptomatic or had AIDS-related complex but not AIDS, had received ZDV for at least 16 weeks and for a median of 13.9 months, and were then switched to ddI had fewer OIs than those who remained on ZDV, although there was no survival benefit up to the date of analysis (Kahn, Lagakos, Richman et al., 1992). Another study supports a similar switch in patients who have not previously had ZDV therapy or have taken and tolerated ZDV for 16 or fewer weeks (NIAID, 1993b). These results may support a strategy of changing antiretroviral therapy prior to clinical or immunologic evidence of failure of initial ZDV therapy. In spite of these studies, however, criteria as to when to change one antiretroviral drug for another are not clear. Studies are needed to clarify this issue and to provide guidance to clinicians and consumers.

The use of a combination of antiretroviral agents is also under intense investigation. A study of a small number of patients indicated that the combination of ZDV and ddC maintains CD4 lymphocyte counts better than ZDV alone (Meng, Fischl, Boota et al., 1992). Other ongoing studies compare ZDV and ddI as single agents with combinations of ZDV with ddI and ZDV with ddC. Results of a recent clinical trial show that in patients who had received prolonged ZDV therapy, the addition of ddC, in contrast to monotherapy with either agent, was associated with delayed HIV disease progression (NIAID, 1993b). However, these results were only observed in patients with CD4 counts between 150 and 300 cells/μl and primarily in those who were clinically symptomatic; thus, additional research is needed. Other combinations of antiretroviral agents with different modes of action, as well as alternating regimens of antiretroviral agents, are under study.

It should be noted that a panel convened by NIH in 1993 developed more detailed guidelines (Sande, Carpenter, Cobbs et al., 1993) for antiretroviral therapy for adults with early HIV infection. Although the guidelines developed by this NIH panel are, in general, consistent with the recommendations presented here, both panels relied often on expert opinion in interpreting the limited existing data. Therefore, the need to discuss options with patients and individualize treatment decisions is emphasized.

Using CD4 Cell Count to Time Initiation of PCP Prophylaxis

Recommendation: Prophylaxis for PCP should be initiated if any of the following conditions are met: (1) the CD4 cell count is < 200 cells/µl (supported by evidence); (2) there has been a prior episode of PCP (supported by evidence); and/or (3) oral candidiasis or constitutional symptoms such as unexplained fevers are present (suggested by evidence).

Recommendation: Oral trimethoprim-sulfamethoxazole (TMP-SMX) is the preferred agent for PCP prophylaxis. (Supported by evidence)

PCP is the most common HIV-associated pneumonia (Murray, Garay, Hopewell et al., 1987). It is associated with significant morbidity and mortality (Haverkos, 1984; Kales, Mullen, Torres, and Crocco, 1987). One of the most encouraging developments in the care of HIV-infected individuals has been the determination of the population at risk and the identification of several agents that are effective in the prevention of PCP.

The panel recommends prophylaxis for PCP in individuals with CD4 lymphocyte counts <200/µl, those with prior episodes of PCP, or those who have specific constitutional signs and symptoms (CDC, 1992c). The goal of PCP prophylaxis is to minimize the number of episodes of PCP in patients at significant risk and to avoid toxicity from unnecessary medications in those not at significant risk for PCP. It is recognized that PCP can occur in patients with CD4 counts >200 cells/µl but at a lower frequency. In addition, CD4 counts can be highly variable, as described above. Because of this variability, some providers routinely begin prophylaxis when the CD4 count falls below 250 cells/µl.

Other clinical indications for initiation of PCP prophylaxis include unexplained fevers and oral candidiasis. A patient with rapidly declining CD4 counts should have CD4 testing more frequently. In such cases, prophylaxis might be initiated at a somewhat higher CD4 level (CDC, 1992c).

There are numerous regimens for PCP prophylaxis, including those described below.

Trimethoprim-Sulfamethoxazole. Oral TMP-SMX has been proven to be the most effective preventive drug in both primary and secondary prophylaxis for PCP. A recent study comparing TMP-SMX with aerosol pentamidine demonstrated that TMP-SMX was significantly more effective in preventing recurrences of PCP (Hardy, Feinberg, Finkelstein et al., 1992). This has been confirmed in a second study conducted in Australia (Carr, 1992). A recent randomized prospective study also supported the superiority of TMP-SMX to aerosolized pentamidine in primary prevention (i.e., in patients with CD4 counts <200 cells/μl and no prior PCP) (Schneider, Hoepelman, Schattenkerk et al., 1992.)

Dose. A variety of dosing regimens of TMP-SMX have been used. At present, the most commonly used dose is one double-strength tablet (sulfamethoxazole, 800 mg per day, and trimethoprim, 160 mg per day). The first study of oral TMP-SMX for primary prophylaxis was performed with one double-strength tablet given two times per day (Fischl, Dickinson, and La Voie, 1988). Other published studies have used one double-strength tablet given one or two times per day, 2 or 3 days per week, but these were not prospective randomized studies (Carr, 1992; Ruskin and LaRiviere, 1991). A study comparing one single-strength to one double-strength tablet of TMP-SMX given daily with aerosolized pentamidine for primary PCP prophylaxis demonstrated that both doses of TMP-SMX were equally efficacious and superior to aerosolized pentamidine (Schneider, Hoepelman, Schattenkerk et al., 1992). Ongoing prospective studies are exploring different dosing regimens of TMP-SMX.

Advantages. TMP-SMX is readily available, inexpensive relative to other agents, and given systemically. Preliminary evidence that TMP-SMX may offer some protection against cerebral toxoplasmosis also supports its use (Carr, Tindell, Brew et al., 1992).

Disadvantages. A substantial number of patients will not be able to tolerate TMP-SMX due to pruritus, rash, myelosuppression, and transaminase elevations (Fischl, Dickinson, and La Voie, 1988). Desensitization may be useful and is currently being evaluated (White, Haddad, Brunner, and Sainz, 1989). Individuals who cannot tolerate high dose TMP-SMX for treatment of PCP may tolerate the low doses used in prophylaxis.

Monitoring. Patients should stop taking the medication and notify their health care provider if they develop a rash, severe gastrointestinal symptoms, or other symptoms suggesting intolerance to the drug. Laboratory work should be individualized but usually includes periodic monitoring of blood counts.

Aerosolized Pentamidine. Aerosolized pentamidine is effective and well tolerated for prophylaxis (Hirschel, Lazzarin, Chopard et al., 1991; Leoung, Feigal, Montgomery et al., 1990). A common regimen is 300 mg given once per month with the Respirgard® II jet nebulizer. When the Fisons ultrasonic nebulizer is used, the dose is 60 mg every

2 weeks after an initial loading regimen of five doses over the first 2 weeks. It is important to use a dose-nebulizer combination that has documented effectiveness.

Advantages. Aerosolized pentamidine is well-tolerated with proven efficacy in people with HIV infection. There are few systemic side effects. Inhalation is monthly and thus is convenient for patients.

Disadvantages. Aerosolized pentamidine is a less effective agent than TMP-SMX in both primary and secondary prophylaxis, and the expense is significantly greater than with other regimens (Freedberg, Tosteson, Cohen, and Cotton, 1991). It requires special equipment and space for delivery. In addition, several reports support a possible increased risk of extrapulmonary pneumocystis in patients receiving aerosolized pentamidine (Northfelt, Clement, and Safrin, 1990; Schneider, Hoepelman, Schattenkerk et al., 1992). Other side effects include persistent cough and bronchospasm (Hardy, Feinberg, Finkelstein et al., 1992).

Administration of aerosolized pentamidine with its potential to induce cough may increase the risk for spread of TB. In light of this, all patients should be evaluated for TB by medical history, tuberculin skin test, chest x-ray, and evaluation of sputum, if clinically indicated, prior to the initiation of aerosolized pentamidine therapy. Aerosolized pentamidine should be administered to patients with TB only under strict adherence to published guidelines. Health care workers administering aerosolized pentamidine should take appropriate precautions (CDC, 1990).

Dapsone. Oral dapsone has been widely used for prophylaxis against PCP (Martin, Cox, Beck et al., 1992; Metroka, Braun, Josefberg, and Jacobs, 1988). A variety of doses and regimens have been used, including 50-100 mg per day. Studies are in progress to document the efficacy of daily and intermittent doses of dapsone compared with TMP-SMX and aerosolized pentamidine in primary and secondary prophylaxis. Some clinicians prefer using dapsone over aerosolized pentamidine in patients who cannot tolerate TMP-SMX, given the increasing concerns about transmission of unrecognized TB and the risk of extrapulmonary pneumocystis. Daily dapsone, when combined with weekly pyrimethamine, has recently been demonstrated to be equally effective in primary prevention of PCP as aerosolized pentamidine (Girard, Landman, Gaudebout et al., 1993).

Advantages. Dapsone is inexpensive, well-tolerated, and systemically absorbed.

Disadvantages. Side effects, including skin rash, fever, and gastrointestinal symptoms, are the most common adverse effects of dapsone. Hemolysis can occur in patients from certain ethnic backgrounds with glucose-6-phosphate dehydrogenase (G6PD) deficiency.

Patients at risk should be screened for this condition. Methemoglo-binemia is a possible complication of dapsone therapy.

Monitoring. Patients should discontinue medications and inform their provider if any symptoms or signs of toxicity develop. Laboratory monitoring should be individualized.

Recommendations for Pregnant Adults and Adolescents

Recommendation: In HIV-infected pregnant women, CD4 counts should be determined on presentation for prenatal care or, for women who have received no prenatal care, at delivery. (Expert opinion)

Recommendation: If the count is >600 cells/μl, the count need not be repeated during pregnancy, unless indicated by clinical symptoms. If the count is <200 cells/μl, it may be repeated every 3 months in order to monitor antiretroviral therapy or initiate new preventive therapies. If the count is between 200 and 600 cells/μl, it should be repeated each trimester. (Suggested by evidence)

The current recommendation of the American College of Obstetricians and Gynecologists (ACOG) is that CD4 counts should be followed every trimester (ACOG, 1992). It is not known how or whether this will alter clinical management. Because of the additional considerations of cost and availability, the panel believes that a CD4 count of 600 cells/μl or greater need not be repeated during pregnancy unless a clinical indication for retesting arises or future studies support it.

Recommendation: HIV-infected pregnant women with CD4 counts <500 cells/μl should be offered antiretroviral therapy with ZDV. They should be informed regarding both the benefits of early therapy with ZDV in asymptomatic HIV-infected patients, as well as potential risks to the fetus. (Suggested by evidence)

The use of ZDV in the management of adults with early HIV infection is discussed in detail above. The benefits and risks to the mother and fetus of ZDV therapy during pregnancy have not been well defined, although its probable utility has been demonstrated in nonpregnant adults with CD4 counts <500 cells/μl. Increased morbidity has been reported in HIV-infected pregnant women with CD4 counts <200 cells/μl (Minkoff, Nanda, Menes, and Fikrig, 1987). Pharmacokinetic studies conducted in three pregnancies documented transplacental passage of the drug and subsequent anemia in two of the infants (Watts, Brown, and Tartaglione, 1991). Subsequent studies did not demonstrate such a high rate of anemia for infants whose mothers received ZDV during pregnancy (O'Sullivan, Boyer, Scott et al., 1992; Sperling, Stratton, O'Sullivan et al., 1992).

Published data showed no fetal malformations in the analysis of 43 pregnant women exposed to ZDV (Sperling, Stratton, O'Sullivan et al., 1992). Although these study populations are small, they currently provide the only information available that addresses this issue. Ongoing trials may clarify the role of ZDV therapy in maintaining maternal health, affecting rates of perinatal HIV transmission, and causing possible toxicity in the fetus. Clearly, more data are needed which are specific to pregnant women with HIV infection. Pregnant women should be provided with information regarding available clinical trials and encouraged to participate.

ZDV is given in the dosage currently used for all adults. The use of other antiretroviral agents during pregnancy has not been studied.

Recommendation: HIV-infected pregnant women should receive prophylaxis for PCP according to the regimen prescribed in this guideline for all adults. (Suggested by evidence)

Because of the lack of information specifically related to PCP prophylaxis during pregnancy, current recommendations are similar to those for the nonpregnant adult. The effects of specific medications used for PCP prophylaxis on the fetus must be taken into consideration, as discussed below.

TMP-SMX is the recommended drug of choice for PCP prophylaxis during pregnancy. Trimethoprim is known to cross the placenta and reaches similar levels in the mother and fetus (Briggs, Bodendorfer, Freeman, and Yaffe, 1983). Although a theoretical risk of teratogenicity exists, no known cases of fetal anomalies can be attributed to its use during pregnancy. A theoretical risk of kernicterus exists for sulfamethoxazole use during pregnancy, but no cases were reported in the current literature. The recommended dose of TMP-SMX is similar to that recommended for nonpregnant adults.

Aerosolized pentamidine has been used for the prevention of PCP infection during pregnancy. Negligible serum levels of pentamidine achieved after aerosol administration would make it unlikely to pose a threat to the fetus (Conte, Chernoff, Feigal et al., 1990).

Dapsone is an alternative for pregnant women who experience side effects with, or are intolerant of, TMP-SMX or pentamidine. Dapsone has been used safely in pregnant women with leprosy (Kahn, 1985).

Testing and Preventive Therapy for Tuberculosis

TB has re-emerged as a major public health threat in the United States, particularly in areas where HIV infection is prevalent (Selwyn, Hartel, Lewis et al., 1989: Sunderam, McDonald, Maniatis et al.,

1986). The dramatic rise in the number of people with active TB has occurred in concert with the HIV epidemic. Although the TB epidemic has not been caused directly by HIV, immunosuppression caused by the virus permits TB infection to progress to active disease at an accelerated pace.

HIV-infected individuals who have been infected with *Mycobacterium tuberculosis* are more likely to develop active TB than those who are not HIV infected. Whereas an HIV-uninfected person with *M. tuberculosis* infection has a 10 percent lifetime risk of developing active TB, an HIV-infected person with *M. tuberculosis* infection has a 10 percent annual risk (Selwyn, Hartel, Lewis et al., 1989). In a population of anergic injection drug users, a significantly higher incidence of TB occurred in HIV-infected individuals than in HIV-uninfected individuals (Selwyn, Alcabes, Hartel et al., 1992). A study of HIV-infected individuals from Spain also demonstrated that anergic patients as well as tuberculin-positive patients had a high risk of development of TB, especially in injection drug users (Moreno, Baraia-Etxaburu, Bouza et al., 1993). Recent data from outbreaks of TB also indicated that immunocompromised persons with HIV are more likely to develop acute primary TB following new infection with *M. tuberculosis* than are individuals without HIV infection (Daley, Small, Schecter et al., 1992).

Three features of TB differentiate it from other OIs that occur during the course of HIV infection. First, because it is spread via the airborne route, it is readily communicable to others. Second, the diagnosis and clinical management of TB in individuals with HIV infection differ from those in individuals who are not infected with HIV. Finally, unlike many OIs that occur in HIV-infected individuals, TB is preventable and may be curable if detected and treated promptly. For all of these reasons, TB merits special focus during the initial evaluation of people with HIV infection.

The distinction between TB infection and active disease (active tuberculosis) must be emphasized. Although active TB may occur at any time in the course of HIV infection, in this section of the guideline, the focus is on the evaluation and management of *M. tuberculosis* infection. The specifics of preventive therapies and methods for early detection of TB infection are discussed. The treatment of active TB in people living with HIV, including details of regimens and isolation procedures, are outside the purview of this document but are discussed in guidelines from the Centers for Disease Control and Prevention (CDC, 1989 and 1992d).

It must be noted that HIV-infected infants and children are at high risk of developing rapidly progressive TB (Khouri, Mastrucci, Hutto et al., 1992; McSherry, Berman, Aguila et al., 1992). Recommendations for adults with TB apply, for the most part, to HIV-infected infants, children, and adolescents, but diagnosis and drug dosage schedules will need to be modified. Future HIV guidelines will need to specifically examine the diagnosis and management of TB in HIV-infected infants, children, and adolescents.

Algorithm 4 (Appendix A) summarizes the following recommendations and discussion. Appendix B-3 details drugs and dosages discussed in this section.

History and Physical Examination

Recommendation: The medical history for all HIV-infected individuals should include:

1. **Assessment of previous TB infection or disease, past treatment or preventive therapy, and history of exposure to *M. tuberculosis*.**

2. **Assessment of the risk for TB infection, including predisposing social conditions (e.g., household contacts, country of origin, homelessness, alcoholism, substance use, history of incarceration, residence in a congregate living situation).**

3. **Assessment of suggestive symptoms (e.g., cough, hemoptysis, fever, night sweats, weight loss). During physical examination, the provider should seek findings indicative of active disease, such as abnormal pulmonary signs or documented weight loss. (Suggested by evidence)**

Recommendation: The medical history for all HIV-infected individuals should also include an assessment of health and social conditions that may affect an individual's ability to complete a course of therapy, specifically, a record of failure to keep medical appointments, homelessness, alcoholism, mental illness, and substance use. (Suggested by evidence)

The comprehensive evaluation of the HIV-infected individual should include: (1) the history of previous infection with TB, (2) prior anti-TB therapy, (3) exposure to household or other close contacts with infectious TB, and (4) the likelihood of exposure to other individuals with TB. Settings where exposure is especially likely to occur include congregate living facilities, such as homeless shelters, prisons, chronic care facilities, and health care settings where outbreaks have been reported. Efforts should be made to complete the history through the acquisition of past medical records and relevant laboratory information. This information may guide the decision to initiate preventive therapy in patients who are anergic and should prompt rapid empiric therapy in individuals with unexplained pulmonary disease (CDC, 1991b and 1992e).

Clinicians performing the clinical history and physical examination should pay particular attention to pulmonary and constitutional signs and symptoms, specifically cough, hemoptysis, fever, night sweats, and weight loss. Presence of these symptoms and signs will influence decisionmaking for both preventive therapy and treatment.

PPD Screening for *M. tuberculosis* Infection

Recommendation: Sequence and timing of testing and evaluation:

1. **All HIV-infected individuals, including those who have received bacille Calmette-Guerin (BCG) vaccination, should be screened using purified protein derivative (PPD) screening for infection with *M. tuberculosis* during their initial evaluation.**

2. **All HIV-infected individuals should be screened for anergy using two control antigens in addition to PPD during their initial evaluation.**

3. **All HIV-infected individuals who are PPD positive or anergic should receive a chest x-ray and clinical evaluation. HIV-infected individuals who have symptoms suggestive of TB should receive a chest x-ray regardless of their PPD or anergy status.**

4. **PPD and anergy testing should be repeated annually in persons who are neither PPD positive nor anergic on initial evaluation. However, persons who reside in areas where TB prevalence is high should be tested every 6 months.**

5. **All PPD-negative or anergic HIV-infected individuals who are exposed to others with suspected or confirmed TB should be immediately tested with PPD and anergy antigens. Repeat testing should be performed in 3 months. (Suggested by evidence)**

Recommendation: Methods for testing and evaluation:

1. **PPD testing should be performed by the Mantoux method. Following intradermal injection of 0.1 ml 5 TU (tuberculin unit) PPD (intermediate strength), the reaction should be assessed after 48 to 72 hours by a trained observer. Reactions of 5 mm or greater induration should be considered positive in persons with HIV infection, regardless of prior BCG vaccination.**

2. **Two of the following three antigens should be used for anergy testing: candida, mumps, or tetanus toxoid. Any degree of induration observed in response to intradermal injection of these antigens constitutes a positive reaction, indicating that the individual is not anergic. (Suggested by evidence)**

PPD testing is the globally accepted method for diagnosis of TB infection. Universal standardization of the PPD tuberculin reagent permits reliable interpretation of testing data. Large population-based studies conducted during the past 50 years have revealed that induration reactions of 10 mm or greater are unlikely to include false-positive tests (Snider, 1982). Although reactions between 5 and 10 mm may include false-positive tests because of infection with nontuberculous mycobacteria (Hanson and Reichman, 1989), CDC elected to use a reaction size of 5 mm or greater for the diagnosis of *M. tuberculosis* infection in all individuals with HIV (CDC, 1986). This criterion was adopted to improve the ability of the test to identify more HIV-infected individuals for preventive therapy. The appropriateness of this strategy is confirmed by a recent study (Johnson, Coberly, Clermont, and Chaisson, 1992). Although results of one study support using a reaction size of 2 mm or greater, these results are based on statistical comparisons that utilize assumptions of population prevalence without confirmation of disease in individuals (Graham, Nelson, Solomon et al., 1992). Thus, currently no evidence supports the use of a smaller reaction size (less than 5 mm) for determination of a positive PPD test.

Results of one study that utilized a decision-analytic approach suggest that PPD testing may be unnecessary prior to initiation of isoniazid (INH) therapy (Jordan, Lewit, Montgomery, and Reichman, 1991). However, the panel did not weigh these results heavily. Because the bulk of the literature emphasizes the importance of PPD testing,, the panel concludes that PPD screening is appropriate. It is important to stress that skin tests should be performed and read at the recommended interval by a trained individual.

PPD testing should likewise be performed in HIV-infected individuals who have received BCG vaccination. Results should be interpreted in the same manner as for all other HIV-infected individuals. Recent data do not support the use of two-stage PPD booster testing in the evaluation of HIV-infected patients (NIAID, 1993c).

Testing for Cutaneous Anergy

Absence of a reaction to the PPD test does not exclude the diagnosis of TB infection but may reflect cutaneous anergy. For this reason, interpretation of a negative PPD test in a person with HIV infection requires conduct and interpretation of anergy testing to determine if the PPD is truly negative (Banerjee, Cromwell, and Furth, 1989; Blatt, Donovan, Freeman et al., 1991; Canessa, Fasano, Lavecchia et al., 1989; CDC, 1991b; Cohen and Nardell, 1990; Graham, Nelson, Solomon et al., 1992; Robert, Hirschel, Rochat, and Deglon, 1989; Zeballos, Cavalcante, Freire et al., 1989). Although false-negative or anergic reactions may occur in approximately 10 percent of the general population (CDC, 1991b), rates of anergy in persons with HIV-associated immunosuppression are higher. Actual rates vary according to the degree of immunosuppression, from approximately 10 percent in asymptomatic individuals with early HIV infection to nearly 60 percent in those with less than 200 CD4 cells/μl (Blatt, Donovan, Freeman et al., 1991).

All persons with HIV infection should receive anergy testing together with PPD testing at the time of initial evaluation. The panel supports anergy testing using two of the following three antigens by the Mantoux method: candida, mumps, or tetanus toxoid. Any degree of induration observed in response to intradermal injection of 0.1 ml of any of these antigens constitutes a positive test. Limitations of the multipuncture anergy skin test devices have been discussed elsewhere (CDC, 1991b). If the patient reacts to any of the anergy test antigens used, then a negative PPD test result usually excludes infection with *M. tuberculosis*. PPD testing should be repeated yearly, with routine anergy screening if the PPD was negative previously. If an individual has been anergic in the past, repeat skin testing with PPD should not be performed except after exposure to TB (Blatt, Hendrix, Butzin et al., 1993).

A patient who does not react to any of the anergy antigens is considered anergic. A negative PPD test result does not exclude the diagnosis of TB infection in the presence of anergy. In anergic patients the clinical evaluation should focus on the identification of active, or infectious, TB.

Chest X-Rays

Recommendation: Chest x-rays should be performed in all HIV-infected individuals who are PPD-positive or anergic or have signs or symptoms suggestive of TB to exclude the presence of active pulmonary TB. If the chest x-ray is normal, see the following recommendation. If the chest x-ray reveals any abnormality, multiple sputum smears and cultures should be performed. If a sputum smear is positive, the patient should be started on anti-TB therapy immediately, pending culture results. Acid-fast bacillus (AFB) isolation should be initiated promptly to reduce transmission to others if the patient is coughing. If the sputum smears are negative, and there is no other etiology for the abnormal chest x-ray, bronchoscopy should be performed, and empiric anti-TB therapy should be initiated, pending the results of the mycobacterial culture. AFB isolation for coughing patients should be maintained until the diagnosis is clarified by smear or culture. In many of these clinical scenarios, diagnostic evaluation and management will need to be individualized, and consultation with an infectious disease or pulmonary specialist may be necessary. (Suggested by evidence)

Several studies demonstrated the variability of the radiographic presentation of pulmonary TB in HIV-infected individuals. Atypical presentations occur commonly, whereas classic apical cavitary disease occurs less often (Goodman, 1990; Long, Maycher, Scalcini, and Manfreda, 1991; Noronha, Pallangyo, Ndosi et al., 1991; Pitchenik and Rubinson, 1985). Instead, pulmonary infiltrates may be interstitial or lobar, often involving multiple segments of the lung. The most common finding in these series is hilar or mediastinal adenopathy without pulmonary infiltrate.

Although highly unlikely in HIV-seronegative individuals, cases of active TB with normal chest x-rays have been documented in HIV-infected individuals (Goodman, 1990; Long, Maycher, Scalcini, and Manfreda, 1991; Pitchenik and Rubinson, 1985). In such cases, it is necessary to rely on other diagnostic methods. Treatment decisions will depend on the following: (1) the results of sputum smears and cultures, (2) clinical presentation, (3) a confirmed history of exposure to TB, and (4) a history of untreated, old TB disease. In HIV-infected individuals, extrapulmonary TB is more common than in individuals who are not HIV infected, occurring in up to 70 percent of individuals with CD4 counts less than 200/μl (Sunderam, McDonald, Maniatis et al., 1986). If fever, weight loss, or night sweats occur in the presence of a normal chest x-ray, diagnostic evaluation should include AFB smears and culture from blood and other sites depending on signs or symptoms.

Sputum Culture

Sputum culture remains the gold standard for diagnosis of pulmonary TB. At least three cultures are needed to maximize sensitivity. Results from cultures are often delayed, requiring up to 8 weeks for final results. New culture and identification systems have shortened the time for identification to within 3 weeks. Newer laboratory techniques are currently under investigation, including polymerase chain reaction (PCR) testing of sputum specimens, which would reduce the time even further (Eisenach, Sifford, Cave et al., 1991). Currently, no reliable serologic test for diagnosis of TB is available. The development and testing of these newer diagnostic methods continues to be an important priority for future research (Grange, 1989; Mattar, Broquetas, Gea et al., 1990; Saad, Kritski, Werneck, and Fonseca, 1990).

For the present, AFB sputum smears offer the advantage of rapid laboratory diagnosis but may not be positive in all cases of pulmonary TB. In individuals who have TB but not HIV infection, the sensitivity of AFB sputum smears is approximately 80 percent. The diagnostic sensitivity of the smear decreases to 66 percent in patients with HIV infection. Thus, mycobacterial sputum cultures are always needed to confirm the presence or absence of pulmonary TB (Collins, 1991;

Long, Scalini, Manfreda et al., 1991) and to exclude atypical mycobacteria. Further studies are needed to evaluate whether induction of sputum improves diagnostic sensitivity.

Preventive Therapy

Recommendation: Preventive therapy for TB should proceed according to the following protocol: (a) regardless of the patient's age, INH preventive therapy should be initiated and continued for 12 months in all HIV-infected individuals who have a positive PPD test and do not have active disease; and (b) preventive therapy should be strongly considered for anergic patients who are known contacts of patients with TB and for anergic patients belonging to groups in which the prevalence of TB infection is at least 10 percent. Specifically, these groups are injection drug users, prisoners, homeless persons, persons living in congregate housing, migrant laborers, and persons born in foreign countries with high rates of TB. Clinicians should consider factors specific to their geographic areas, including the incidence and prevalence of TB infection, when making the decision to start preventive therapy. (Suggested by evidence)

Isoniazid preventive therapy should be initiated in all HIV-infected individuals who have a positive PPD test but do not have evidence of active TB, regardless of age (CDC, 1990). Oral doses of 300 mg per day or 900 mg two times per week may be used for adults and adolescents. Infants and children should receive INH at a dose of 10-15 mg/kg per day (maximum 300 mg per day) (CDC, 1986).

Pyridoxine therapy at oral doses of 50-100 mg per day may be useful for prevention and treatment of INH-induced peripheral neuritis in patients with inadequate nutritional intake (CDC, 1986).

Patients should be educated concerning signs and symptoms of clinical liver disease, which may result from INH-associated hepatotoxicity. Baseline serum liver enzymes (ALT or AST) should be performed on all patients before initiation of INH therapy. Mild to moderate elevation in liver enzymes is not a contraindication to initiation of INH preventive therapy. If symptoms of liver disease occur, liver enzymes should be repeated. Monitoring should occur more frequently in patients with elevated baseline values and in those with underlying liver disease. Consultation with an infectious disease or pulmonary specialist may be necessary.

Recommendation: In persons with HIV who are exposed to drug-resistant strains of *M. tuberculosis,* an alternative preventive therapy should be considered. Consultation with a pulmonary or infectious disease specialist should be sought. In addition, the presence of AFB

on sputum smear should prompt immediate empiric anti-TB therapy tailored to community drug susceptibility patterns, pending final determination of drug susceptibility testing. (Suggested by evidence)

Strains of *M. tuberculosis* resistant to multiple antibiotics, including INH, rifampin, ethambutol, and streptomycin, have been isolated with increasing frequency in the United States, especially in New York City and Miami (Edlin, Tokars, Grieco, and Crawford, 1992; Fischl, Uttamchandani, Daikos et al., 1992). For individuals who have been exposed to *M. tuberculosis* in areas where multidrug-resistant TB (MDR-TB) has been reported, the likelihood of exposure to these strains should be ascertained. Factors associated with an increased possibility of transmission include: (1) the degree of infectiousness of the source case, as manifested by active cough and/or AFB-positive sputum; (2) the closeness and intensity of exposure to MDR-TB; and (3) susceptibility for development of active TB following exposure. Persons with HIV infection are at enhanced risk for development of disease following exposure to *M. tuberculosis* and should be considered candidates for prophylaxis against MDR-TB if exposure is considered likely. If exposure to MDR-TB is suspected, consultation with public health and local experts should be obtained. Guidelines for assessment of risk and proposed agents for use in these circumstances are available (CDC, 1992e).

Completion of the prescribed course of anti-TB preventive therapy is essential to prevent the development of disease and the emergence of resistance to the antibiotics used for treatment. Issues concerning patients' adherence to treatment regimens and recommendations for improving adherence are presented in "Improving Adherence to Tuberculosis Regimens" in this chapter.

Recommendation: The evaluation and management of *M. tuberculosis* infection in pregnant women should be performed as described in the previous recommendations. Preventive INH therapy is not contraindicated in pregnant women and should be initiated according to the recommendations above. In asymptomatic women, chest x-rays should be performed only after the first trimester, and a lead apron shield should be used. In women with symptoms suspicious for TB, x-rays should be performed with a lead apron shield irrespective of stage of pregnancy. (Suggested by evidence)

Studies have demonstrated that PPD testing and chest x-rays are both reliable and safe for use with pregnant women, if appropriate precautions are taken (Bonebrake, Noller, Loehnen et al., 1978; Montgomery, Young, Allen, and Harden, 1968; Present and Comstock, 1975; Swartz and Reichling, 1978; Weinstein and Murphy, 1974). INH has been widely used during pregnancy without undue sequelae (Good, Iseman, Davidson et al., 1981; Lowe, 1964; Schein-horn and Angelillo, 1977). Coadministration of pyridoxine with INH is recommended in pregnant women in order to provide supplementa-tion to the mother and prevent neurotoxicity in the fetus (Atkins, 1982; Snider, Layde, Johnson, and Lyle, 1980; Warkany, 1979).

Improving Adherence to Tuberculosis Regimens

The previous section outlined testing and preventive therapy for TB in persons with HIV infection. Individuals with TB who do not complete their therapy have an increased probability of relapse, dis-ability, or even death. Additionally, at potentially large social cost, these individuals may infect others and may develop drug-resistant strains of *M. tuberculosis* (CDC, 1992e).

Failure to complete TB treatment has been shown to be a common problem (Alcabes, Vossenas, Cohen et al., 1989; CDC, 1992d; Combs, O'Brien, and Geiter, 1990; Werhane, Torbeck, and Schrufnagel, 1991). For example, a study in 1988 from a large urban hospital found that only 11 percent of 178 patients with TB completed their therapy. The remaining 89 percent did not return for outpatient followup and failed to renew medication necessary to complete therapy. Consequently, 27 percent of the discharged individuals were later readmitted with TB (Brudney and Dobkin, 1991).

A variety of studies have shown that completion of therapy can be facilitated by improved communication between the health care provider and patient, simplified treatment regimens, and improved followup (CDC, 1989, 1992d, and 1993). This section discusses approaches that can promote completion of therapy and increase patient adherence to treatment. Several of these recommendations will require the concerted action of both public and private agencies. Providers should check with their local health departments about the availability of public health nursing staff to work with reluctant patients or those with complicated cases.

Recommendation: TB prophylaxis and treatment regimens should be closely monitored by health care providers to ensure completion of the entire course of therapy. (Suggested by evidence)

Methods for monitoring the course of therapy include: (1) assess-ing clinical and microbiologic response to treatment, (2) interviewing patients, (3) reviewing medical records for missed appointments, (4) monitoring drug levels, and (5) counting returned pills. Several methods used in combination may provide the best results. For example, a provider may check for drug metabolites in urine and also ask the patient if he or she has been taking medications regularly.

Recommendation: Providers should use the simplest appropriate anti-TB regimen and educate their patients about the importance of completing the full course of anti-TB therapy. (Expert opinion)

The first step in the education process is to identify the patients' concerns about their disease and medications. Barriers to completion of treatment, including lack of access to drugs, inadequate transportation, confusion caused by neurologic complications of illnesses, and lack of child care, should be identified. To foster the completion of treatment, the provider should take time to determine how new medication will fit into the patient's lifestyle and other treatment regimens and to explain the need for this therapy to the patient. Specific steps include:

1. Writing a list of medications (name, dose, and scheduling).

2. Involving family members and friends in the treatment process.

3. Using intermittent drug therapy.

4. Using fixed-dose combinations of drugs.

5. Providing specially labeled and designed packages for medication.

6. Providing educational materials that are written in the patient's language and are at an appropriate literacy level.

7. Using electronic beepers or other devices when available to remind patients of their medication schedules.

Research also has indicated that successful treatment occurs more often when patients have an identified provider. For this reason, the same provider or team of providers should see patients on repeat visits.

Recommendation: Case management and directly observed therapy (DOT) should be used when needed to ensure successful completion of anti-TB therapy. (Expert opinion)

Case management should be made available to HIV-infected individuals receiving anti-TB therapy. Case managers can identify and overcome barriers to completion of therapy through the identification, procurement and coordination of services (see Chapter 5, Case Management for Persons Living With HIV). In addition, an intensive form of treatment followup, DOT, is an effective method of ensuring completion of therapy. DOT involves a "hands-on" approach in which an outreach worker or other health care provider observes all medications taken by the patient. DOT may be performed at a clinic or at locations convenient to the patient such as the patient's home or a drug treatment program. State regulations, however, vary considerably regarding who is allowed to administer medications. Additionally, the effectiveness of DOT may be enhanced by using patient incentives such as meals, subway tokens, and clothes.

DOT programs should be provided, when possible, through existing programs and service delivery systems, including HIV clinics, drug treatment centers, and community-based agencies. Although both case management and DOT can be very effective at increasing adherence, each requires extensive health care resources. Specifically, services and medications should be available at minimal or no cost, located in places easily accessible at convenient times, and provided by specially trained staff.

Recommendation: Community members and recognized community leaders should be involved in the development and implementation of public health responses to TB. (Expert opinion)

An often overlooked source of information about health and social needs in a community at risk for TB are community members themselves. The CDC has recommended the following tasks for community coalitions: defining problems and identifying obstacles related to excessive TB rates; establishing health goals and realistic objectives; determining priorities; and developing, implementing, and evaluating strategies (CDC, 1992d). Within these tasks, identifying adherence barriers and developing programs to overcome these barriers should be emphasized.

Testing and Treatment of Syphilis

Syphilis and HIV infection are epidemiologically associated. The incidences of both infections have risen dramatically over the past 10 years, and coinfection is not uncommon (Gregory, Sanchez, and Buchness, 1990; Haas, Bolan, Larsen et al., 1990; Hicks, Benson, Lupton, and Tramont, 1987; Johns, Tierney, Felsenstein, 1987; Katz and Berger, 1989; Lukehart, Hook, Baker-Zander et al., 1988; McLeish, Palido, Holland et al., 1990; Radolf and Kaplan, 1988; Tikjob, Russel, Petersen et al., 1991). When syphilis occurs in the immunocompetent individual, its diagnosis and treatment are relatively straightforward; however, coinfection with HIV may alter the natural history, laboratory diagnosis, and response to therapy of syphilis (Hook, 1989; Musher, Hamill, and Baughn, 1990). It is crucial for the provider to be aware of the potential for these alterations when evaluating and treating syphilis in the HIV-infected person.

This section provides recommendations for assessment and treatment of syphilis in HIV-infected adults and adolescents. The recommendations are summarized in Algorithm 5 (Appendix A). Issues specific to syphilis evaluation and management in HIV-infected pregnant women are presented in "Special Recommendations for Pregnant Women" in this section.

Diagnosis

Recommendation: All HIV-infected adolescents and adults should be evaluated for syphilis by conducting a thorough medical history, a physical examination, and serologic testing. The medical history should include: (a) a review of previous syphilis infection or disease, including history of past treatment; (b) a review of posttherapy serologic followup; and (c) history of lumbar punctures (LPs). (Suggested by evidence)

Because HIV and syphilis frequently occur together (Katz and Berger, 1989), the panel recommends that all patients with HIV infection be evaluated for syphilis.

In terms of history-taking, providers should be aware that patients often cannot give precise answers to all questions. Efforts should be made to complete the history through acquisition of past medical records, as details of the history may affect interpretation of syphilis serologic test results and subsequent management decisions.

In addition, sexually experienced adolescents have the highest rates of sexually transmitted diseases (STDs) of any age group (Bell and Hein, 1984). Therefore, a sexual history with screening pelvic or genital examination and laboratory assessment are indicated for even asymptomatic adolescents who have had sexual intercourse.

Recommendation: The initial serologic screening for current or past syphilis should be performed with nontreponemal tests (rapid plasma reagin [RPR] or Venereal Disease Research Laboratories [VDRL]). All reactive nontreponemal tests should be followed by a specific treponemal test (microhemagglutination assay for *Treponema pallidum* [MHA-TP] or fluorescent treponemal antibody absorption [FTA-ABS]). (Suggested by evidence)

Recommendation: In patients with clinical findings suggestive of syphilis who have nonreactive nontreponemal tests, serum should be diluted to overcome the possibility of a prozone phenomenon due to high antibody levels. (Suggested by evidence)

Recommendation: In primary syphilis, both nontreponemal and treponemal serologic tests may be nonreactive. Therefore, if primary syphilis is suspected, dark-field microscopy and direct fluorescent antibody staining for *T. pallidum* (DFA-TP) from a scraping of suspected lesions should be performed. If a dark-field examination cannot be done and primary syphilis is suspected, empiric treatment should be instituted. (Suggested by evidence)

In persons without HIV infection, the VDRL and RPR (nontreponemal tests) and the FTA-ABS and MHA-TP (treponemal tests) are highly sensitive for primary and secondary syphilis, particularly when used in combination (i.e., a nontreponemal with a treponemal test) (Jaffe, 1984). Although the specificity of these tests (separately and in combination) is also usually high, it may be reduced for patients with other acute and chronic conditions such as Lyme disease, leprosy, or malaria (Hook and Marra, 1992). For patients with suspicious lesions, confirmatory testing for syphilis includes dark-field microscopy and DFA-TP.

In persons with HIV infection, the laboratory diagnosis of syphilis may be complicated. Some case studies and case series reported that serologic results in HIV-infected patients are similarly valid as results in noninfected patients (Musher, Hamill, and Baughn, 1990). Other case studies and a cross-sectional study reported results of nonreactive or lower-than-expected titers on both nontreponemal and treponemal serologic tests in persons with both HIV and syphilis (Gregory, Sanchez, and Buchness, 1990; Haas, Bolan, Larsen et al., 1990; Hicks, Benson, Lupton, and Tramont, 1987; Tikjob, Russel, Petersen et al., 1991). Such results suggest that the alteration of immune regulatory function or the immunosuppression caused by HIV infection may interfere with serologic reactivity. In fact, the cross-sectional study, which examined reactivity on treponemal tests over time in persons with a confirmed history of syphilis, showed an association between declining reactivity and decreasing CD4 counts (Haas, Bolan, Larsen et al., 1990). Conversely, a retrospective chart review (Hutchinson, Rompalo, Reichart, and Hook, 1991) described individuals with syphilis and HIV who had higher serologic titers than a group of non-HIV-infected patients, controlling for stage of syphilis. Such elevated titers may result from the high levels of antibodies to cardiolipin antibody often found in HIV-infected patients. It should be noted that high levels of cardiolipin antibody may also result in the prozone phenomenon and a false negative assay.

Because this evidence is inconsistent and no data were derived from randomized trials or epidemiologic studies, no generalizable conclusion is possible regarding the sensitivity and specificity of serologic testing for syphilis in HIV-infected persons. Although the clinical experience of the panelists suggests that serologic testing is typically accurate in HIV-infected patients, the panel acknowledges the inconsistency reported in the literature and the biologic plausibility of altered serologic reactivity in immunocompromised individuals. The panel thus believes that there is a need for clinicians to individualize the interpretation of serologic test results for syphilis in the HIV-infected patient, as recommended above and discussed further below.

First, because of the association between HIV infection and syphilis, the presumption should be made that a positive nontreponemal serology represents a true infection and should always be followed by confirmatory testing with treponemal tests. Second, when suspicious lesions exist and confirmatory testing using dark-field microscopy cannot be done, empiric treatment should be instituted (Briggs and Paavonen, 1984). This proviso includes situations in which suspected lesions are located in the mouth. For such lesions, dark-field microscopy is not suitable because of the presence of other oral spirochetes (Tramont, 1990). Direct florescence antibody staining also may not be reliable in oral lesions due to possible cross reactivity with other oral treponemes (Schuster and Schuster, 1990). In addition, chancroid and herpes simplex ulcers can mimic syphilitic lesions.

Management

Recommendation: Evaluation of the cerebrospinal fluid (CSF) for evidence of neurosyphilis may be prudent for all HIV-infected individuals with positive treponemal serologies. (Suggested by evidence) Specifically, CSF evaluation should be discussed with and encouraged in all HIV-infected individuals with primary, secondary, or latent syphilis, or infection of unknown duration. (Expert opinion)

This recommendation reflects the panel's synthesis of: (a) evaluation of the published evidence for the recent reappearance of neurosyphilis, particularly in persons coinfected with HIV; (b) evaluation of the published evidence regarding the possibility of an accelerated course of syphilis in HIV-infected individuals, potentially resulting in a comparatively high incidence of asymptomatic neurosyphilis in these individuals; (c) consensus that the knowledge obtained from an LP influences treatment choice (i.e., the patient with asymptomatic neurosyphilis, if diagnosed, will receive therapy appropriate for neurosyphilis, whereas the same patient, if undiagnosed, may receive inadequate therapy); and (d) evaluation of the advantages and disadvantages of more aggressive diagnostic and treatment approaches. The following discussion describes the relevant published literature and elaborates on the panel's interpretation of the literature.

Before 1980, the occurrence of neurosyphilis in young persons and its development early in the course of syphilis were extremely rare. Since the identification of HIV infection, many cases of neurosyphilis have been identified in coinfected persons who are young or at an early stage of syphilis (Musher, Hamill, and Baughn, 1990). These findings suggest that HIV infection accelerates or otherwise alters the natural history of syphilis, with an important outcome being the early and virulent onset of neurosyphilis.

The virtual nonexistence of early cases of neurosyphilis in the 1950s, 1960s, and early 1970s is supported by the results of an extensive search of the literature and interviews with three generations of syphilologists

(Musher, Hamill, and Baughn, 1990). It likewise appears from this review that the recent upsurge of neurosyphilis cases is seen specifically in persons coinfected with HIV. A retrospective cohort study (Katz and Berger, 1989) found that 44 percent of their neurosyphilis patients had AIDS. (It is unclear whether more patients had less advanced or asymptomatic HIV infection.) A followup study (Lukehart, Hook, Baker-Zander et al., 1988) found that, although there were no significant differences in how often treponemes were isolated from the CSF of HIV-infected and noninfected patients, there was significantly more cerebrospinal leukocytosis in those participants with HIV infection. This finding may indicate additional, albeit culture negative, neurosyphilis in the HIV-infected group. Finally, a cross-sectional study (Holtom, Larsen, Leal, and Leedom, 1992) estimated the prevalence of asymptomatic neurosyphilis to be 1 percent in a consecutive sample of outpatient clinic patients with HIV infection, irrespective of syphilis serologic status. This estimate most likely represents a minimum for the following reasons:

■ It does not include possible neurosyphilis in those who refused LP or were lost to followup (about the same proportion of the coinfected population as underwent LP).

■ It did not consider the potential for treatment failure and consequent asymptomatic neurosyphilis in those who had recent treatment for syphilis (those having had any treatment for syphilis in the past 6 months were excluded).

■ It only counted reactive CSF VDRL tests as indicative of asymptomatic neurosyphilis (any other type of abnormalities found in the CSF were excluded).

Nonetheless, in those who were coinfected and received LPs, a prevalence of 9.1 percent of reactive CSF VDRL tests were found. Like the 1 percent prevalence estimated for the study's overall HIV-infected population, this 9.1 percent is most likely an underestimate.

Several additional studies and reports in the literature discussed the hypothesis of an accelerated or more florid course of syphilis in HIV-infected persons. These include a retrospective record review (Hutchinson, Rompalo, Reichart, and Hook, 1991), a prospective cohort study (Gourevitch, Selwyn, Davenny et al., 1993), and several case studies and series (Gregory, Sanchez, and Buchness, 1990; Johns, Tierney, and Felsenstein, 1987; McLeish, Palido, Holland et al., 1990; Radolf and Kaplan, 1988; Tikjob, Russel, Petersen et al., 1991). All of the case reports describe unusual presentations of syphilis in HIV-infected persons. Both the retrospective record review (Hutchinson, Rompalo, Reichart, and Hook, 1991) and the cohort study (Gourevitch, Selwyn, Davenny et al., 1993) directly compared syphilis stage at presentation in HIV-infected individuals with that in uninfected individuals. Both studies found no difference in stage at presentation of syphilis in HIV-infected and uninfected persons. However, neither study examined syphilis stage at presentation while controlling for stage of HIV infection or CD4 count in the HIV-infected group. It is possible that differences in syphilis stage of presentation for persons with varying stages of immune function were obscured by assessing HIV-infected persons as a single group.

Although the studies described above are variously flawed (usually by small sample sizes and suboptimal sampling schemes), a consistent theme appears to suggest higher than expected rates of neurosyphilis in persons with HIV infection. The apparent association of HIV infection and neurosyphilis over time adds weight to this suggestion. What remains unclear is whether this finding is due to an accelerated course of syphilis in coinfected individuals, the failure of conventional treatment for early syphilis and subsequent relapse in these individuals, or the level of HIV-associated immune suppression in the individual with syphilis infection which may affect host response to treponemal invasion or to treatment.

The followup study discussed earlier (Lukehart, Hook, Baker-Zander et al., 1988), which found no difference between individuals with and without HIV infection in how often the CNS was invaded in early syphilis, reported that conventional treatment for early syphilis did not clear the CNS of coinfected individuals, whereas more aggressive treatment did. This result, although based on very small numbers of patients, suggests that treatment decisions for the coinfected individual are best made after either excluding or recognizing asymptomatic neurosyphilis. (Additional discussion of treatment issues in early syphilis appears below in the recommendations.) The panel feels that the information provided by LPs is particularly important in determining appropriate treatment for coinfected individuals with secondary or later stages of syphilis, in which dissemination of treponemes has most likely occurred. It should be noted that treponemal serology may remain reactive for life, and therefore results of this assay should be interpreted in the context of the patient's medical history.

Finally, the panel considered carefully the disadvantages associated with performing LPs (including issues of risk, discomfort, cost, varying patient preferences, and the uncertainties inherent in interpreting results of LPs in HIV-infected persons), as well as the advantages of early LP (including the opportunity to identify early neurosyphilis and prevent the onset of symptoms through the use of appropriate treatment). The panel concluded that a prudent medical approach, such as that recommended above, is warranted. However, confirmatory research, which examines the necessity of such an approach, is needed.

Recommendation: If neurosyphilis is excluded, primary, secondary, early latent, and late latent syphilis, as well as infection of unknown duration, should be treated with three intramuscular (IM) doses of benzathine penicillin per week, 2.4 million units. (Suggested by evidence)

Using information obtained through a review of articles about the evolution of syphilis treatment and cure in non-HIV-infected patients, Musher, Hamill, and Baughn (1990) deduced that the currently recommended dosage for treatment of primary and secondary syphilis (a single dose of benzathine penicillin, 2.4 million units) lies just on the margin of adequacy. Although this dosage has been effective in treating syphilis in non-HIV-infected individuals, it has remained possible to, on occasion, recover treponemes from such patients subsequent to treatment. The effectiveness of this treatment may be dependent on intact host immune function. Clearly, in HIV-infected individuals with compromised immune function, the validity of the prior assumption should be questioned.

In fact, several case studies and case series documented the failure of conventional treatment for primary and secondary syphilis to clear the CSF of HIV-infected persons and thus prevent relapse in these persons (Berry, Hooton, Collier, and Lukehart, 1987; Gregory, Sanchez, and Buchness, 1990; Johns, Tierney, and Felsenstein, 1987). A case-control study (Telzak, Greenberg, Harrison et al., 1991) which examined success and failure of syphilis treatment in HIV-infected and uninfected persons with primary and secondary syphilis (treatment regimens not specified) showed lower rates of treatment success in HIV-infected patients, controlling for stage of syphilis. (Treatment success was defined as four-fold or greater RPR decline within 6 months for primary syphilis or within or after 6 months for secondary syphilis.) Although this study was limited in a variety of ways, these results and those of the case reports are consistent with the need for a different, perhaps more aggressive, treatment regimen for the earlier stages of syphilis in coinfected persons.

A prospective cohort study (Gourevitch, Selwyn, Davenny et al., 1993) compared responses to treatment in a cohort of HIV-infected and uninfected injection drug users in a methadone treatment program. Only two patients in the cohort (one HIV infected, one uninfected) in the earlier stages of syphilis (primary, secondary, and early latent) received standard (one dose of benzathine penicillin) therapy. Therapy was successful in both of these patients. Thirteen patients in the same stages of syphilis (10 HIV infected, 3 uninfected) received more aggressive treatment of between two and four doses of benzathine penicillin; treatment again was successful in all of the patients regardless of HIV status. Although the investigators concluded that these results suggest that there is no difference in response to treatment between HIV-infected and uninfected individuals, the important issue of which treatment schedule is more effective for coinfected individuals in the earlier stages of syphilis cannot be addressed because of the small number of patients who received the standard therapy. In fact, the distribution of treatment schedules across study participants suggests that there is a distinct preference among providers to prescribe more aggressive treatment (perhaps particularly for coinfected individuals or individuals at high risk for HIV infection), rather than to err on the side of potentially less adequate, but simpler, regimens.

Therefore, the panel feels the evidence is sufficiently suggestive of conventional (one dose of benzathine penicillin) treatment failure in HIV-infected patients with primary, secondary, and early latent syphilis to justify a more aggressive approach to treating these patients. Such an approach seems additionally appropriate given the benign nature of the treatment. The panel therefore recommends the more intensive treatment approach described above, with the overarching goal of minimizing the chance of relapse or progression to neurosyphilis. However, confirmatory prospective studies of success rates using different treatment schedules should be a critical priority for future research.

Recommendation: HIV-infected individuals with abnormal CSF findings (presence of cells, increased protein, or positive VDRL test results) should be treated with a regimen effective against neurosyphilis: intravenous aqueous penicillin, 2-4 million units every 4 hours for 10 to 14 days. (Suggested by evidence)

Recommendation: Treatment for presumptive neurosyphilis should be encouraged when CSF cannot be evaluated. (Expert opinion)

In light of: (a) the potential for syphilis to develop into neurosyphilis early in the course of infection in persons coinfected with HIV, (b) the above discussion regarding the possibilities of conventional treatment failure and relapse, (c) the impact of LP results in treatment discrimination, and (d) the seriousness of relapse and neurosyphilis, the panel believes that the prudent approach is to encourage patients to accept treatment for presumptive neurosyphilis when CSF is not evaluated. The panel recognizes the practical issues in the treatment of neurosyphilis including the need for hospitalization or multiple outpatient visits, as well as the limitations of current data which preclude conclusions regarding optimal regimens.

Patients who refuse intravenous treatment can be treated with procaine penicillin, 2.4 million units per day IM for 10 days, plus 500 mg probenecid orally four times per day. A recent study on neurosyphilis treatment in HIV-infected persons showed that ceftriaxone at 1-2 g IM per day (no difference was found between 1 and 2 g) may be a viable alternative treatment in patients who refuse standard therapy (Dowell, Ross, Musher et al., 1992). It should be noted, however, that the failure rate for this treatment was approximately the same as that for procaine penicillin, approaching 20 percent. Indeed, further studies of effectiveness are needed, including clinical trials which compare treatments.

Recommendation: Patients with syphilis and a reported reaction to penicillin should be referred to an allergist or infectious disease specialist for further management. (Expert opinion)

There are no proven alternative therapies to penicillin for the treatment of neurosyphilis, congenital syphilis, and syphilis in pregnancy. Therefore, when true penicillin allergy is suspected, consultation with a specialist is recommended.

Monitoring

Recommendation: All HIV-infected individuals should have a nontreponemal serologic test for syphilis performed at least annually. In addition, serologic tests should be performed after exposure to, or diagnosis of, any STD. (See also the recommendation for syphilis testing in pregnant women.) (Expert opinion)

Recommendation: In HIV-infected individuals who have been diagnosed with and treated for syphilis, followup nontreponemal serologies should be performed at posttreatment intervals of 1, 2, 3, 6, 9, and 12 months following treatment and annually thereafter. The same test should be used consistently because titers are not comparable between different nontreponemal tests. (Expert opinion)

Following treatment, titers should decrease by four-fold in 6 months for primary and secondary syphilis (CDC, 1988). Titers that increase, do not decline sufficiently, or remain unchanged may signify reinfection or inadequately treated disease. Patients should be reevaluated, including evaluation of the CSF, and retreated as appropriate. Potential confounding of serologic tests as a result of concurrent HIV infection should be considered, as described in the recommendations.

Recommendation: HIV-infected individuals diagnosed with syphilis should be evaluated for other STDs and substance use and managed accordingly. The diagnosis of syphilis and other STDs in HIV-infected individuals should alert the provider to counsel the patient on the

importance of safe sex practices. (See Disclosure Counseling by Providers in Chapter 1.) (Expert opinion)

Substance use has been epidemiologically associated with HIV infection (CDC, 1988; Quinn, Cannon, and Glasser, 1990). Thus, it is important to provide patients with information regarding available resources for substance use treatment.

Special Recommendations for Pregnant Women_____

Recent data have demonstrated the resurgence of congenital syphilis in selected urban centers in the United States (New York City Department of Health, 1989). This finding highlights the importance of the early recognition and appropriate treatment of syphilis in pregnant women.

Recommendation: HIV-infected pregnant women should be screened for syphilis with a nontreponemal test (RPR or VDRL) at entry into prenatal care, during the third trimester, at delivery, and if the patient is exposed to or presents with symptoms or signs of a STD. (Suggested by evidence)

Pregnant women should be evaluated for syphilis in conjunction with entry into prenatal care or at delivery, as these visits represent an opportunity to provide screening and treatment. In addition, evaluation during the third trimester is crucial if treatment is to be completed in time to reliably prevent congenital syphilis.

Recommendation: Treatment and followup of syphilis is the same for pregnant women as for nonpregnant adults. For treatment to reliably prevent the sequelae of congenital syphilis, penicillin therapy must be completed at least 4 weeks before delivery. All infants born to women with syphilis should be assessed for congenital syphilis and managed as appropriate. (Supported by evidence)

The therapy for syphilis during pregnancy is designed to provide effective treatment to the mother and prevent congenital infection of the fetus (New York City Department of Health, 1989). Oral therapies such as erythromycin or tetracycline and its derivatives may provide adequate therapy for the mother but do not effectively treat the fetus (CDC, 1988). In addition, tetracyclines have adverse effects on the teeth and bones of the fetus and should not be used during pregnancy (Kline, Blatter, and Lunin, 1964). Penicillin is the only therapy that is known to be effective for both mother and fetus.

Oral Examinations

Some of the earliest published work describing AIDS included descriptions of oral lesions found in persons with HIV infection (Feigal, Katz, Greenspan et al., 1991; Greenspan, Barr, Sciubba et al., 1992; Greenspan, Greenspan, Conant et al., 1984; Greenspan, Greenspan, Lennett et al., 1985; Pindborg, 1989; Scully, Laskaris, Pindborg et al., 1991). In addition, some HIV-infected persons may have an unusually rapid and destructive periodontal disease (Masouredis, Katz, Greenspan et al., 1992; Tenenbaum, Mock, and Simor, 1991; Winkler, Murray, Grassi, and Hammerle, 1989). Because HIV-infected individuals experience these unique oral conditions in addition to dental problems common to all individuals, both specialized as well as routine oral care are required by individuals with HIV infection. Despite this need, many persons with HIV infection have poor access to any dental care (Capiluto, Piette, White, and Fleishman, 1991).

Oral lesions may provide the only early indication of HIV infection and are important in the classification of the stage of HIV disease (Greenspan, Greenspan, Overby et al., 1991; Melnick, Engel, and Truelove, 1989; Schulten, Reinier, and Van der Waal, 1990). In an otherwise asymptomatic individual, recognition of the presence of oral lesions, such as oral candidiasis and/or hairy leukoplakia, may be crucial for some therapeutic decisions and indicate progression of disease (Katz, Greenspan, Westenhouse et al., 1992). In addition, oral lesions may be used as part of a staging system for HIV progression and as endpoints in clinical drug trials (Royce, Luckman, Fusaro, and Winkelstein, 1991). Although oral lesions have been seen in all groups at risk for HIV infection, most published work described studies in men (Bolski and Hunt, 1988; Feigal, Katz, Greenspan et al., 1991). As yet, only a small body of literature concerns women (Shiboski, Greenspan, Westenhouse et al., 1992; Tukutuku, Muyembe-Tramfun, Kayembe, and Ntumba, 1990) and children (Davis, 1990; Katz, Mastrucci, Leggott et al., in press; Ketchem, Berkowitz, McIlveen et al., 1990; Leggott, Robertson, Greenspan et al., 1989; Palumbo, Jandinski, Connor et al., 1990).

The panel's recommendations for oral examinations are based largely on published literature (Sheiham, 1977; Preventive Services Task Force [US], 1989); however, the recommendation for optimal timing of oral examinations is based on clinical judgment.

Recommendation: Oral examinations should be performed by the primary care provider during every physical examination. (Expert opinion)

Recommendation: All oral mucosal surfaces should be carefully examined. The HIV-infected individual should be informed of the importance of oral care and educated about common HIV-related oral lesions and associated symptoms. (Suggested by evidence)

Recommendation: HIV-infected individuals should have a dental examination performed by a dentist at least two times per year. With the appearance of oral lesions or problems, more frequent dental followup is necessary. (Suggested by evidence)

Recommendation: Primary care providers and dentists should be trained to identify and treat oral lesions associated with HIV infection. Any HIV-infected individual with unusual or suspicious lesions should be referred to an appropriate specialist. (Expert opinion)

The published literature consistently supports the importance of the recognition of oral lesions in HIV-infected individuals. It is therefore important that at each contact with the primary care provider, an oral examination is performed. These routine examinations may be performed by a range of health care providers (Feigal, Katz, Greenspan et al., 1991; Katz, Greenspan, Westenhouse et al., 1992; Melnick, Engel, and Truelove, 1989), including primary care physicians, physician assistants, and nurse practitioners who have been adequately trained in oral examination and diagnosis. Ideally, such training should include seminars incorporating slides of lesions and led by trained examiners with clinical experience; in addition, primary care providers should take opportunities to discuss HIV-related oral care with dentists.

Routine oral examinations should include careful inspection of the oral soft tissues, with particular attention paid to the soft palate and lateral margins of the tongue. Any soft tissue changes, as well as periodontal disease and the presence of caries or defective restorations, should be noted. Information about the importance of oral care should be made available as part of this examination. The HIV-infected individual should be instructed to report symptoms such as oral pain, dryness, bleeding, difficulty in swallowing, change in taste, and loosening of teeth. Many oral lesions require the expertise of a dentist for correct diagnosis and management (Scully, Laskaris, Pindborg et al., 1991). Referral may need to be made to a specialist such as a dentist trained in oral medicine, periodontology, or oral surgery (Masouredis, Katz, Greenspan et al., 1992).

Few published studies define the appropriate timing of dental examinations in any population (Sheiham 1977; Preventive Services Task Force [US], 1989). Therefore, our recommendation for the frequency of examinations by primary care providers and dentists is based on clinical judgment and experience in monitoring other immunologically compromised populations. Routine oral examinations by the primary care provider would detect lesions that may indicate progression of HIV infection. Scheduled dental examinations should be conducted by a dentist at least two times per year. This is consistent with the existing recommendations for non-HIV-infected individuals (Preventive Services Task Force [US], 1989). It is well documented that as immune function declines, the probability of developing oral lesions increases dramatically (Begg, Phelan, Mitchell-Lewis et al., 1992; Katz, Greenspan, Westenhouse et al., 1992). Thus, it is imperative that the frequency of dental examinations be increased as immune function declines.

The goal of these examinations is to identify disease and institute preventive care (Greenspan and Greenspan, 1991; Winkler, Murray, Grassi, and Hammerle, 1989). All providers should be trained in the recognition and treatment of lesions associated with HIV infection, including pseudomembranous candidiasis (thrush) and erythematous candidiasis (Dodd, Greenspan, Katz et al, 1992), hairy leukoplakia due to Epstein-Barr virus (Greenspan and Greenspan, 1991), Kaposi's sarcoma (Ficarra, Person, and Silverman, 1988), aphthous ulcers, ulcers due to herpes simplex virus (Phelan, Eisig, Freedman et al., 1991), oral warts due to papillomavirus (Greenspan, de Villiers, Greenspan et al., 1988), and periodontal disease (Klein, Quart, and Small, 1991; Masouredis, Katz, Greenspan et al., 1992; Swango, Kleinman, and Konzelman, 1992; Winkler, Murray, Grassi, and Hammerle, 1989). Less common lesions include non-Hodgkin's lymphoma, *Mycobacterium avium-intracellular* complex, bacillary angiomatosis, and salivary gland enlargement, as well as ulcers due to varicella-zoster virus, cytomegalovirus (CMV), syphilis, histoplasma, and cryptococcus. Complaints of xerostomia due to treatment with didanosine (dideoxyinosine, ddI) and ulcers due to treatment with zalcitabine (dideoxycytidine, ddC) have been noted (Dodd, Greenspan, Westenhouse, and Katz, 1992).

Eye Examinations

The range of ocular complications associated with HIV disease include: (1) noninfectious microangiopathy, most often seen in the retina, consisting of cotton-wool spots with or without intraretinal hemorrhages and other microvascular abnormalities; (2) opportunistic ocular infections, primarily CMV retinitis; (3) conjunctival, eyelid, or orbital involvement by neoplasms seen in patients with HIV infection (i.e., Kaposi's sarcoma and lymphoma); and (4) neuro-ophthalmic lesions, primarily syphilitic optic neuritis (Insler, 1987; Jabs, Green, Fox et al., 1989). The most frequently encountered lesions are cotton-wool patches, vascular congestion, hemorrhages, chorioretinitis, segmental vasculitis, and pallid papillae (Balacco, Angarano, Moramarco et al., 1990; Freeman, Chen, Henderly et al., 1989).

Recommendation: A careful history of visual disturbances and an eye examination, including funduscopy, should be performed by the primary care provider during the patient's routine visits. Patients should be educated by their provider about the symptoms of CMV retinitis,

including the presence of floaters, and visual disturbances such as blurring and loss. (Expert opinion)

Recommendation: HIV-infected individuals should have an eye examination performed by a qualified eye doctor at least: every 3 to 5 years at ages 20 to 39, every 2 to 4 years at ages 40 to 64, and every 1 to 2 years at ages 65 and over. Examinations should be more frequent if problems develop. (Expert opinion) Patients with any visual symptoms suggestive of CMV should be referred immediately for confirmation of diagnosis by a qualified eye doctor. (Suggested by evidence)

CMV retinitis, the most common OI associated with visual loss in HIV infection, is seen most frequently in patients already diagnosed with AIDS (Association for Research on Vision and Ophthalmology, 1990; Cooney, 1991). An HIV-infected person who is otherwise asymptomatic and has a CD4 cell count >200 cells/μl is at low risk for developing this OI (Fisher, Nussbaum, and Frasier, 1990). Recent data indicate that the median CD4 count at the time of diagnosis of CMV retinitis is <50 cells/μl (Henderly and Jampol, 1991). Another report suggests that the incidence of retinitis is about 25 percent prior to death for HIV-infected patients (Drew, 1992).

Cotton-wool patches are the most frequent lesions found on funduscopic examination (Balacco, Angarano, Moramarco et al., 1990). They are rarely seen, however, in the asymptomatic HIV-infected person with a CD4 count >200 cells/μl. More typically, they appear in advanced stages of HIV infection (Association for Research on Vision and Ophthalmology, 1990).

Few published studies define the appropriate timing of eye examinations in any population. Therefore, our recommendation for the frequency of examinations by primary care providers and qualified eye doctors is based on clinical judgment, experience in monitoring HIV-infected individuals, and existing recommendations for non-HIV-infected individuals (American Academy of Ophthalmology, 1992). Providers often refer patients to a qualified eye doctor for baseline funduscopy when CD4 counts fall below 100 cells/μl because of the increased risk of CMV retinitis at this stage of HIV infection. Further studies are needed in this area, and current trials evaluating the efficacy of prophylactic therapy against CMV retinitis may clarify this issue.

The literature does not provide any data on the value or reliability of eye examinations by the primary care provider in the detection of CMV retinitis. However, since CMV retinitis can be treated by the use of available therapies, it is imperative that this condition be detected as early as possible to avoid vision loss. When eye examinations are conducted as routine parts of primary care visits, in combination with the patient monitoring his or her own visual symptoms, the potential for early identification is maximized. Thus, education of asymptomatic patients with HIV infection regarding signs and symptoms of CMV retinitis, such as floaters (semitransparent bodies perceived to be floating in the field of vision that move rapidly with eye movement but drift slightly when the eyes are still) and blurred or sudden loss of vision (including unilateral vision change or subtle field defects, usually without pain or redness), is a crucial component of the patient's care. Likewise, instructing patients to report such symptoms promptly to their primary care providers is essential for further management by a qualified eye doctor.

Pap Smears

With the increasing impact of the HIV epidemic on women, the evaluation of HIV-associated gynecologic conditions and the provision of appropriate gynecologic care for women with HIV infection have become important areas of concern for the primary care provider. This section addresses issues relating to gynecologic care of women with HIV infection. In particular, we emphasize the importance of regular gynecologic examination as an integral component of primary care. We also emphasize the value of the Pap (cervical) smear as a key component of that care.

Studies of women with non-HIV-associated immunosuppression, including renal transplant recipients and patients with Hodgkin's disease, reported increased rates and severity of cervical abnormalities (Halpert, Fruchter, Sedlis et al., 1986; Rellihan, Dooley, Burke et al., 1990; Sillman, Stanek, Sedlis et al., 1984). Women with HIV-associated immunosuppression appear to be at similar risk. A number of published case reports suggest increased prevalence or severity of cervical disease, as well as a more rapid primary progression of untreated cervical dysplasia to more advanced stages of cervical disease in HIV-infected women (Bradbeer, 1987; Byrne, Taylor-Robinson, Munday, and Harris, 1989; Henry, Stanley, Cruikshank, and Carson, 1989; Maiman, Fruchter, Serur, and Boyce, 1988). In addition, several studies, discussed in detail below, report results consistent with these case reports.

Current methods of evaluating cervical cells include Pap smears, colposcopy with endocervical curettage, directed biopsies, and cone biopsies. However, the optimal timing and relative benefits of these have not been well defined specific to the HIV-infected woman. The following recommendations, summarized in Algorithm 6 (Appendix A), are based on the published literature, in conjunction with panel consensus and the current ACOG recommendations for the routine screening and evaluation of cervical cytologic abnormalities.

It should be noted that invasive cervical cancer has been included as an AIDS-defining diagnosis (CDC, 1992a).

Recommendation: A Pap smear should be performed as part of the complete initial gynecologic examination in all women with HIV infection. For pregnant women, Pap smears should be performed at entry into prenatal care or, for women with no prenatal care, following delivery and prior to discharge. (Suggested by evidence)

Providers in all primary care settings should perform complete gynecologic examinations, including recto-vaginal examinations and Pap smears. Pap smears are recommended for all sexually active adolescents and for women 18 years of age or older. Recent studies have demonstrated that Pap smears are an effective screening test for women with HIV infection (ACOG, 1989). In the general population, the sensitivity of Pap smears is between 50 and 90 percent, with repeat Pap smears leading to dramatic improvements in sensitivity (Wright, 1993).

The panel does not recommend the use of colposcopy as an initial screening test for detection of cervical cytologic abnormalities in HIV-infected women. Only one study compared the concordance of colposcopic results with those of Pap smears in a small number of HIV infected women (Maiman, Tarricone, Vieira et al., 1991). Although results showed that Pap smears yielded a higher rate of false negatives, the study was seriously limited by a nonblind review by the pathologist or colposcopist as to the HIV status of the patients and the lack of a control group of HIV-uninfected women. Conversely, other recent data suggest that the sensitivity of Pap smears in HIV-infected women is approximately 81 percent, within the same range as Pap smear sensitivity in noninfected women (Wright, 1993). Further studies of this issue are needed.

Studies have shown that HIV-infected women have a markedly higher prevalence of abnormal Pap smears than women without HIV infection. In a review of Pap smears of 414 women who underwent HIV testing, abnormal Pap smears (including all types and degrees of abnormalities) were found in 5 percent of 213 uninfected women and 63 percent of 201 HIV-infected women (Provencher, Valme, Avarette et al., 1988). A study comparing prevalence of cervical dysplasia in HIV-infected women attending outpatient facilities with that in noninfected women in the same community found a higher prevalence in those who were HIV infected (Marte, Cohen, Fruchter, and Kelly, 1992). In a study of 77 patients undergoing colposcopy who had abnormal Pap smears at entry, higher grade cytologic abnormalities and more severe histology were found in HIV-infected women than in uninfected women (Maiman, Fruchter, Serur et al., 1990). Another study that compared cervical intraepithelial neoplasia (CIN) in HIV-infected and uninfected women reported a rate of 4.7 percent in uninfected women and 12.5 percent in HIV-infected women (Conti, Muggiasca, and Conti, 1989). An evaluation of women enrolled in a study of heterosexual transmission of HIV found that HIV-infected women had a higher prevalence of cervical and vaginal abnormalities than did uninfected women. This study also showed evidence of higher rates of human papilloma virus (HPV) in HIV-infected women (Schrager, Friedland, Maude et al., 1989). Issues related to this latter finding are explored further below. Finally, in a study of results of cytologic smears of the cervix, 41 percent of women with HIV infection had evidence of dysplasia/neoplasia compared with 9 percent of uninfected injection drug users and 4 percent of outpatient controls (Schäfer, Friedmann, Mielke et al., 1991). Association of these abnormalities with immunosuppression will be discussed below.

These studies are variously limited by small sample sizes, non-blinding of observers, imperfect controls, and differing definitions of cervical cytologic results. Although none of these limitations is uniformly found in all studies, there is strong consistency across results regarding the association between HIV infection and the occurrence of abnormal cervical findings. This consistency suggests the need for gynecologic monitoring of the HIV-infected woman using Pap smears.

Various classification schema for the interpretation of Pap smears have been proposed. Published expert opinion varies in terms of which scheme is preferable. Table 1 presents the two most commonly used schema.

Recommendation: Pap smears should be repeated according to the following schedule: two times in first year; annually when the initial Pap smears are normal; every 6 months when there is a history of HPV infection, previous Pap smear showing squamous intraepithelial lesion (SIL) (see Table 1), or symptomatic HIV infection; after treatment of any cervical lesion or the underlying cause of an inflammation; and if no endocervical cells are seen. (Suggested by evidence)

The recommendation above regarding timing of Pap smears is based on the following:

1. Current established guidelines for frequency of Pap smears in women in the general population (annually or less frequently, at the discretion of the provider).

2. Knowledge that repeating Pap smears dramatically increases the sensitivity of the screen.

3. Understanding that cervical abnormalities are likely to be more common, more severe, and perhaps more rapidly progressive in women with HIV infection, as described above.

4. The potential role of HPV and immunosuppression in mediating cervical abnormalities in HIV-infected women.

Table 1. Suggested classification of squamous epithelial cell cytologic changes

1. Atypical squamous cells of undetermined significance (specify recommended followup and/or type of further investigation).

2. Squamous intraepithelial lesions (SILs): comment on presence or absence of cellular changes consistent with human papilloma virus (HPV) infection:

   ■ Low-grade SIL, encompassing:
      Cellular changes consistent with HPV infection
      Mild dysplasia/CIN 1

   ■ High-grade SIL, encompassing:
      Moderate dysplasia/CIN 2
      Severe dysplasia/CIN 3
      Carcinoma in situ/CIN 3

3. Squamous carcinoma.

---

[1] Summarized from abstract presented at the Workshop on Terminology and Classification of Vaginal Cytology, National Cancer Institute, December 1988.

HPV infection and the degree of HIV-associated immunosuppression may play an important role in the severity and progression of cervical disease. HPV genital infection has been strongly linked to cancer of the genital tract (Durst, Gissmann, Ikenberg, and zur Hausen, 1983). Microbiologic and biochemical evidence of this association was supported by a prospective study of 241 women (Koutsky, Holmes, Critchlow et al., 1992). This study showed a significant association between HPV infection and the incidence and development of CIN. (The highest risk was demonstrated in women infected with HPV types 16 and 18.) HIV-associated immunosuppression may facilitate this pathologic effect of HPV infection on the cervix. Several studies lend support to this hypothesis. A study of 67 women enrolled in a variety of programs found that the risk of abnormal cervical cytology was 42 times higher in women who were coinfected with HIV and HPV than in women with neither infection (Feingold, Vermund, Burk et al., 1990). Women infected with either HIV or HPV were also at increased risk for cervical abnormalities; however, the risk appears to be lower than that for coinfected individuals. Another study suggested a similar pattern of increased risk in coinfected symptomatic women compared with asymptomatic and HIV-seronegative women (Vermund, Kelley, Klein et al., 1991). A study of commercial sex workers in Kinshasa, Zaire, demonstrated that 38 percent of HIV-infected women and 8 percent of uninfected women had HPV DNA in their cervico-vaginal lavage (Laga, Icenogle, Marsella et al., 1992). HIV infection, HPV infection, and CIN were strongly associated.

The severity of immunosuppression may also be an important factor in mediating the risk of cervical abnormalities in women with HIV infection. In the study by Feingold, Vermund, Burk et al. (1990) described above, HPV was increasingly associated with cervical abnormalities in the presence of increasing symptomatology for HIV infection. Another study of 32 HIV-infected women who underwent colposcopy found that 100 percent (5 of 5) of women with AIDS diagnosis had CIN compared with 30 percent in HIV-infected women without AIDS (Maiman, Tarricone, Vieira et al., 1991). Patients with CIN had lower CD4 counts than those with less severe cervical abnormalities, suggesting either a more rapid rate of progression of cervical abnormalities with decreasing immune function or a more severe presentation of disease. In a review of medical records of 73 women attending an HIV clinic, an association between low CD4 counts and abnormal Pap smears was found (Stein, Roche, Mathur-Wagh et al., 1991). A cross-sectional study of 32 HIV-infected women compared HPV prevalence in women with CD4 counts less than 200 cells/μl and women with greater than 200 cells/μl (Johnson, Burnett, Willet et al., 1992). Results showed that HPV was more prevalent in the low CD4 cell group; in addition, HPV types 16 and 18 were more prevalent in that same group. These results suggest a role for the intact immune system in suppressing HPV infection, particularly the more virulent types. Finally, in a study of cervical smears in 111 HIV-infected women, a significant association was found between prevalence and severity of cervical dysplasia with CD4 lymphocyte depletion (Schäfer, Friedmann, Mielke et al., 1991).

Again, although these studies are limited in various ways, including unknown duration of infection with either HIV or HPV, they suggest the need for close monitoring of cervical abnormalities, especially in women with HPV infection or symptomatic HIV infection. Currently, however, there is inadequate information to judge conclusively the costs and benefits of performing Pap smears more than one time per year in HIV-infected women.

Recommendation: All women, including pregnant women, should be referred to a trained clinician for colposcopy when: (1) the Pap smear indicates atypical cells of undetermined significance, (2) the Pap smear demonstrates either low-grade or high-grade SILs or carcinoma, or (3) there is a history of untreated SILs. (Suggested by evidence)

Colposcopy is a useful tool for further assessment of abnormal cervical cytology. Its results were compared with those of conization and hysterectomy, and concordance rates of 67 to 95 percent were reported (Stafl and Mattingly, 1973; Townsend, Ostergard, Mishell, and Hirose, 1970). In addition, reliability of colposcopy markedly improved with increasing experience of the examiner (Briggs and Paavonen, 1984). Therefore, performance of colposcopy should be limited to providers who have received specific training.

Primary care providers should be aware of the indications for colposcopy and should refer their patients to an appropriately skilled professional. The referral should be reserved for individuals with a Pap smear that demonstrates atypical cells of undetermined significance, SIL, or carcinoma. The evaluation should include a visual examination of the vulva, vagina, and cervix; endocervical curettage; and directed (not random) biopsies.

Pregnancy Counseling

Counseling HIV-infected women with regard to reproductive issues and options should be included in any primary care practice. The counseling must focus on the health outcomes that might be expected as a result of any choice, for the mother as well as for the infant. These outcomes include the possible effects of pregnancy on the mother's health and the progression of her HIV infection, the issues pregnancy raises with regard to enrollment in clinical trials and access to new agents, the effect of HIV infection on birth outcome, the risk of HIV transmission from mother to infant, the prognosis of HIV infection in infants, and the issues related to the care of children who have lost their parents. Even with these emphases, pregnancy counseling remains challenging because evidence shows that a woman's decision to become pregnant or to continue or terminate a pregnancy is not related in a straightforward way to the woman's HIV status and possible HIV-related outcomes (Arras, 1990).

Parameters for the Pregnancy Counseling Model_____

Recommendation: Contraceptive, preconception, and prenatal counseling for the woman with HIV should be nondirective, with the focus on the woman and her needs, rather than on the beliefs held by the provider. In addition, counseling should be client-oriented, with the provider listening more than talking. The psychological state of the individual—in particular, the level of anxiety or depression that might be present—should be assessed. The counselor should impart the most recent information, using terms and language that are familiar to the woman being counseled, on possible effects of HIV infection on pregnancy and of pregnancy on HIV infection, the current health status of the woman, transmission rates to the fetus, transmission to sexual partners, and the need for contingency plans for future care of children. (Suggested by evidence)

Based on the general counseling literature, we recommend the following model to assist the primary care provider in counseling HIV-infected women and their families about pregnancy decisions. It is essential that counseling be nondirective and client-oriented and have a psychological as well as an educational focus. Nondirective counseling allows the woman and her needs, interests, and expectations, not the beliefs held by the primary care provider, to become the focus of the dialog. In this scenario, the primary care provider adopts a nonjudgmental approach.

An effective counseling session will be client-oriented, with the provider listening more than talking and not advocating personal opinions or feelings. It is also important to recognize that decisions regarding pregnancy often are not individual decisions; in some cultures, family members play a significant role in decisionmaking (Holman, Berthaud, Sunderland et al., 1989).

The educational dimension of the session(s) should include all of the information needed for making decisions. Topics should include those that every woman, regardless of her HIV status, would consider when making decisions regarding pregnancy, in addition to topics specific to HIV. For example, in counseling women who are interested in contraception, a description of barrier methods such as condoms should include a discussion of their three important advantages: contraception, prevention of HIV transmission to uninfected partners, and reduction of the possibility of reinfection with HIV or infection by another sexually transmitted disease. It is also important to determine whether the woman is able to access care for a pregnancy termination if that is her decision. In addition to these general themes, specific psychological and educational interventions should be part of the counseling session, and these are discussed in the ensuing recommendations.

Nondirective counseling can be led by both trained health care providers and peers (Hutchinson and Kurth, 1991). Sessions can be held for individuals, couples (conjoint counseling), and groups. Neither the length of time required for effective nondirective counseling nor the number of sessions required is discussed in the literature.

Effects of Variables Other than HIV Infection on Pregnancy Decisions

Recommendation: Maternal characteristics (such as age, attitudes and beliefs, general health status, pregnancy history) as well as maternal HIV status should be discussed when a woman is counseled regarding contraception and pregnancy choices. (Suggested by evidence)

Three published studies looked specifically at the role of HIV status in pregnancy continuation decisions. All three studies found that factors other than HIV status were important in the decision about whether to continue a pregnancy. Holman, Berthaud, Sunderland, and colleagues (1989) examined the impact of counseling in a population of women of color. Of the 27 women who learned that they were HIV infected within sufficient time to terminate the pregnancy, only 4 (15%) chose to do so. Another study found that in a methadone clinic, there was essentially no difference when termination rates were compared in HIV-infected and HIV-uninfected women: 50 percent of HIV-infected and 44 percent of HIV-uninfected women elected termination (Selwyn, Carter, Schoenbaum et al., 1989). Finally, in a series of case studies of HIV-infected women, those who carried their pregnancies to term reported that factors unrelated to HIV status were as important as their HIV status in this decision (Christiano and Susser, 1989; Flaskerud and Rush, 1989; James, Rubin, and Willis, 1991). It is noteworthy that these three studies found consistent results across disparate populations.

In terms of general maternal characteristics, it is well documented that extremes of maternal age (younger than 18 and older than 35), independent of HIV status, are related to risk during pregnancy and adverse perinatal outcome. Also well documented are the independent roles of social support and the participation of a woman's partner and/or family in pregnancy choices and outcome (Holman, Berthaud, Sunderland et al., 1989). Although it remains unclear as to how these factors interact with HIV status, psychological and educational counseling must assess these factors common to all women involved in making decisions regarding pregnancy.

There has been some research on how knowledge, attitude, and beliefs about HIV infection affect reproductive decisions. Several studies indicated that there is a range of both understanding and beliefs about the cause and effects of HIV infection, as well as a range of situations and practices (such as psychiatric diagnoses, drug addiction, suicide attempts, prostitution, and incarceration) which affected pregnancy decisions (Christiano and Susser, 1989; Flaskerud and Rush, 1989; James, Rubin, and Willis, 1991). In these studies, the independent role of HIV status in pregnancy decisionmaking is not clear. Based on the above evidence, we recommend that all maternal factors be discussed in conjunction with HIV status during counseling sessions.

Risks Associated with Pregnancy in HIV-Infected Women_____

Recommendation: HIV-infected women should be informed that currently there is no evidence of a direct deleterious effect of pregnancy and childbirth on the progression of early HIV infection. (Suggested by evidence)

The panel found no compelling evidence for a direct deleterious effect of pregnancy on an HIV-infected woman's health or the course of her HIV infection (Minkoff, 1990; Selwyn, Carter, Schoenbaum et al., 1989). Further studies that include large numbers of HIV-infected women, both pregnant and nonpregnant, are needed to fully assess this relationship.

Pregnancy Outcomes in HIV-Infected Women_____

Recommendation: HIV-infected women should be informed that adverse natal outcomes have not been consistently documented in infants of HIV-infected women. (Suggested by evidence)

Four studies from the United States and one from Kenya reported contradictory results regarding maternal HIV infection and infant well-being at birth. Minkoff, Henderson, Mendez, and colleagues (1990) examined birth records of infants born to HIV-infected and HIV-uninfected women and found no correlation between HIV status and either birthweight or APGAR scores. Semprini, Ravizza, Bucceri, and others (1990) sought a potential interaction between HIV status and drug addiction in terms of birth outcome. They concluded that there were no detrimental independent effects of HIV status on perinatal outcomes.

Some results, however, pointed in the opposite direction. Koonin, Ellerbrock, Atrash, and others (1989) examined birth outcomes in women who had died of AIDS and had carried a fetus to term within 1 year before their death. They found negative outcomes in 13 of 16 delivered pregnancies (11 were premature and 2 were stillborn). These findings applied to women in late-stage HIV disease, and it is unclear whether the results can be generalized to pregnancy during early HIV infection. In addition, this study neither included a control group, nor ensured that the sample series was unbiased. Temmerman, Plummer, Mirza, and colleagues (1990) in a large case-control study in Nairobi, Kenya, found an association between maternal HIV infection and adverse obstetric outcome (specifically, low birthweight and stillbirth). It is not clear whether these findings can be generalized to the U.S. population. Although, again, there seems to be consistency across results. Additional research is certainly warranted to study pregnancy outcomes in women with early HIV infection.

Recommendation: HIV-infected women should be informed that the risk of perinatal HIV transmission ranges from 13 to 39 percent. (Supported by evidence)

Several studies report maternal-infant HIV transmission rates ranging from 13 to 39 percent (Blanche, Rouzioux, Moscato et al., 1989; Hutto, Parks, Lai et al., 1991; Ryder, Nsa, Hassig et al., 1989). Multiple factors appeared to influence the rate of HIV maternal-infant transmission, including maternal stage of HIV infection, viral load, and possibly other maternal infections (Feldblum and Fortney, 1988; Koonin, Ellerbrock, Atrash et al., 1989). Twin births were studied to identify the timing and frequency of HIV maternal-infant transmission. A study by Goedert, Duliege, Amos, and colleagues (1991) evaluated the HIV status of twins born to HIV-infected women in nine countries and found that often only one twin was infected, most often the first-born. Infection of the first twin suggests that this occurs in the cervix and birth canal. However, cesarean section cannot be regarded as a preventive measure because a substantial proportion of both first- and second-born twins delivered by cesarean section were infected. This study showed an 11 percent rate of maternal-infant transmission.

Pregnant women with HIV-infection should be encouraged to disclose their HIV status to their providers so that pregnancy can be monitored, the details of the care can be discussed, and the evaluation needed by the child can be planned. (See section on Diagnosis of HIV Infection in Infants and Children in Chapter 4.)

Long-Term Impact on the Family

Recommendation: The long-term implications of pregnancy decisions on the family, including emotional issues related to the loss of a parent or parents and foster care, should be discussed during counseling. Women should be encouraged to discuss these issues with significant others. (Expert opinion)

Pregnancy counseling should include a discussion of potential consequences within the family relating to the loss of a parent or parents. Such consequences may include foster care and the emotional well-being of both HIV-infected and uninfected children. Because the entire family feels the effects of pregnancy decisions, women may benefit from discussing their specific situations with their partners or others who function for them in important support roles.

Decisions Regarding Pregnancy

Recommendation: The decision of the woman with HIV regarding conception and continuation or termination of pregnancy should be respected. (Expert opinion)

This recommendation is a consensus of the panel, based on the synthesis of several areas of literature. First, no compelling evidence exists at this time for a direct effect of pregnancy on a woman's health or the course of her HIV infection. Only two studies have examined the relationships among mothers' HIV status, childbirth outcomes, and mothers' subsequent health status (Feldblum and Fortney, 1988; Koonin, Ellerbrock, Atrash et al., 1989), and neither controlled for stage of HIV infection at the start of pregnancy. The panel thus feels that there is no scientific basis to recommend for or against pregnancy on health-related grounds as they relate to the mother. Second, evidence suggests that approximately one-fourth of infants born to HIV-infected women are themselves infected. Here the panel feels that interpretation and personalization of probabilities are highly individual matters. Third, as discussed above, HIV status is not necessarily the pivotal factor in a woman's decisionmaking regarding conception or pregnancy continuation. Finally, through discussion of long-term consequences of pregnancy decisions on the family, the HIV-infected woman can consider her needs alongside those relating to the future of the family. The panel believes that no provider can or should assume the responsibility for persuading a woman to shift her priorities, once she has made a decision.

Breast-Feeding

Recommendation: Breast-feeding is not recommended for HIV-infected mothers in the United States. (Suggested by evidence)

A recent decision analysis based on available data focused on different settings and compared mortality associated with breast-feeding and not breast-feeding in infants born to mothers with and without HIV infection (Hu, Heyward, Byers et al., 1992). The analysis showed that in populations with a high prevalence of HIV infection and approximately equal overall infant mortality for breast-fed and non-breast-fed infants (usually settings in which clean water and adequate nutritional options are available), breast-fed infants born to HIV-infected mothers had higher mortality than those not breast-fed. The analysis also showed that for populations in which, overall, breast-feeding is protective of infants (i.e., mortality is lower in infants who are breast-fed, typically where there is only limited access to clean water and nutritional options), breast-fed infants born to HIV-infected mothers maintained lower rates of mortality than those not breast-fed. Our recommendation considers these results in light of conditions in the United States, where there is access to clean water and adequate food and nutritional formulas (Oxtoby, 1988). Thus, breast-feeding is not recommended for HIV-infected mothers in this country.

Access of Women with HIV Infection to Clinical Trials and Investigational Treatments

Minorities, women, adolescents, and injection drug users were not enrolled in the HIV-related clinical trials of the mid-1980s, reflecting in part the early demographics of the HIV epidemic (Cotton, 1990; Fauci, 1989; Levine, 1986; Svensson, 1989). However, despite the increasing numbers of women, minorities, adolescents, and injection drug users affected by HIV infection, there has been a lag in their enrollment in clinical trials. Although access has been limited for each of these groups for a variety of reasons (El-Sadr and Capps, 1992; Fauci, 1989; Lagakos, Fischl, Stein et al., 1991), this section specifically examines the reasons behind, and consequences of, the underrepresentation of women in HIV-related clinical trials. It focuses first on non-pregnant women of childbearing age and then on pregnant women. It concludes by suggesting strategies that individual providers and patients may employ to make optimal use of existing treatment options.

As women of childbearing age constitute one of the fastest growing segments of the AIDS population, limited access for women to HIV-related clinical trials and investigational treatments has serious implications (CDC, 1992f). These include restricting the understanding of the pharmacokinetics, safety, and efficacy of alternative interventions for women and, in the case of individual patients, narrowing the range of potential therapeutic options. In addition, access to investigational treatments by women of childbearing age is a complex and multidimensional issue that is influenced by public and organizational policy, provider perception, and women's social roles. These factors are tightly interwoven and superimposed on the traditional need to balance the risks and benefits of participation in a specific clinical trial.

Important strides in public policy have been made recently that should facilitate greater inclusion of women in clinical trials. NIH has codified (Public Health Law 103-23) an earlier policy calling for inclusion of women in research studies in numbers proportionate to their number in the affected population(s) (NIH, 1993). The NIH statement requires that where such inclusion is not possible, the reasons be well-justified (NIH, 1991). In addition, FDA has issued an update of its guidelines for clinical research on women (FDA, 1993), which encourages the inclusion of women of childbearing age in clinical trials in order to provide further understanding of the effect of these agents on women. Until this update, the FDA guidelines recommended against including women of childbearing potential from participation in early phase studies of most drugs except when the drug was intended as a life-saving or life-prolonging measure (FDA, 1977).

71

A substantial effort has been made to include in clinical trials under-represented populations such as women, minorities, adolescents, and injection drug users. In 1989, NIAID established the Community Programs for Clinical Research on AIDS (CPCRA) to involve community-based providers and their patients in clinical trials (NIAID, 1991). Also since 1989, the National Institute of Child Health and Human Development (NICHD) has funded 28 sites to conduct clinical trials in HIV-infected, predominantly minority children, adolescents, and pregnant women in collaboration with the AIDS Clinical Trials Group (ACTG) program. In addition, the ACTG recently developed programs targeting certain populations, particularly women and adolescents.

In spite of these initiatives in public policy and the availability of new programs for clinical trials and investigational treatments, women have faced, and continue to face, significant access barriers. These include the woman's role as caregiver for family and children, as well as cultural and economic barriers (El-Sadr and Capps, 1992). At the level of the individual provider and research institution, and across all phases of research, the increased requirements involved when women participate (such as pregnancy testing, additional paperwork, the disenrollment of women who become pregnant, the cost of child care, etc.) have limited the enrollment of women in studies. Finally, clinicians—lacking information on the effects of investigational agents in HIV-infected women of childbearing age—have been hesitant to prescribe antiretrovirals and other HIV-related treatments even after their approval (Minkoff and DeHovitz, 1991; Minkoff and Moreno, 1990).

Since the vast majority of women contracting HIV infection are in their childbearing years, it is not surprising that many become pregnant at some point during the course of their illness. Thus, the issue of pregnant women's access to clinical trials and investigational treatments is germane to the larger issue of women's access to those trials.

From a scientific perspective, the study of investigational drugs in pregnant women is crucial because of the potential specific effects of pregnancy on treatment, including changes in hormonal levels and volume of distribution of drugs. In addition, studies are necessary to obtain safety data for the pregnant woman and her infant and to determine the effect of the drug on maternal-infant HIV transmission. This information is of vital importance prior to approval of a drug and its subsequent use in pregnant women.

The 1993 FDA guideline update on women in clinical trials does not address the difficult question of women who are already pregnant or who become pregnant (Merkatz, Temple, Sobel et al., 1993). However, it should be noted that under the old FDA guidelines, pregnant women could be granted access to experimental drugs under life-threatening circumstances, and this type of access remains available under the new guidelines (FDA, 1977). In addition, exceptions to treatment restrictions may be attempted through various mechanisms available under the treatment IND (investigational new drug) regulations or expanded access processes.

Policymakers, pharmaceutical companies, researchers, and clinicians have been and are concerned about the potential adverse effects of investigational treatments on the fetus (Bennett, 1993; Levine, 1991; Levine, Dubler, and Levine, 1991; Nolan, 1990). However, from a legal standpoint, according to the American Civil Liberties Union, basic principles of law protect the manufacturers of new and investigational drugs from strict liability for harm caused by an investigational drug as long as they have adequately informed and obtained consent from study participants (Hunter, 1992). This protection from liability provided by current tort law should diminish fears when weighed against the significant need for additional research related to women and HIV infection.

Guidelines for conducting clinical trials are urgently needed to address the issue of the inclusion of pregnant women and their access to investigational drugs. These guidelines should avoid *a priori* exclusion of pregnant women and should specify an approach that includes assessment of stage and gravity of the disease; specific drug characteristics, including risks associated with the drug; phase of the proposed study; and availability of other treatment options. The involvement of the pregnant woman in these assessments is essential and should include sufficient information so that she can make an informed decision regarding participation. In addition, policymakers should encourage pharmaceutical companies to conduct relevant safety studies.

It is crucial to recognize the key role of individual providers in terms of facilitating the access of women with HIV infection to investigational treatments. With proper information, providers can assess the risks and benefits of specific treatments alongside the needs of individual patients. Providers who care for women with HIV infection can increase access by:

- Seeking information regarding clinical trials available in the community by calling 1-800-TRIALS-A.

- Linking women to settings that offer appropriate investigational treatments.

- Engaging women in discussions of the risks and benefits of participation in specific trials or undergoing specific investigational treatments.

- Providing opportunities for ongoing patient education and dialog.

- Developing referral networks with local CPCRA, NICHD, and ACTG programs and other clinical trial programs.

- Joining with and offering case management services, which include coordination of care, child care, etc.

- Pursuing the treatment IND and expanded access processes when appropriate.

3 Guideline: Caring for Adolescents with Early HIV Infection

Introduction

HIV infection is spreading rapidly in the adolescent population. AIDS cases among adolescents have increased by 77 percent over the past 2 years (House Select Committee, 1992). Since 1988, AIDS has been the sixth leading cause of death among 15- to 24-year-old individuals in the United States (Novello, 1993).

The prevalence of HIV infection in adolescents varies by geographic location and age. A seroprevalence survey of teenage applicants to U.S. military service showed that the prevalence of HIV infection ranged from less than 0.1 per 1,000 in the North Central States to more than 2 per 1,000 in urban counties of Texas and the East. The overall prevalence for teenagers in this survey was 0.34 per 1,000 (Burke, Brundage, Goldenbaum et al., 1990). In youth enrolled in the U.S. Job Corps, the overall prevalence of HIV infection was found to be 3.6 per 1,000. Seroprevalence was highest in minority youth from large northeastern cities (St. Louis, Conway, Hayman et al., 1991). Rates as high as 160 per 1,000 HIV-infected older adolescents (18-21 years) were found in a study of a New York City homeless shelter (Stricof, 1991). Given the long latency period between infection and AIDS-defining illnesses, most individuals diagnosed with AIDS under 30 years of age were probably infected as adolescents.

Caring for adolescents with early HIV infection presents a unique set of issues: differences in the epidemiology of HIV infection among youth; variable laws and practices regarding consent and confidentiality for minors under the age of 18; special barriers to receiving HIV care; lack of availability of age-specific clinical services; special features of the progression of HIV infection during adolescence; limited standards for routine management of HIV-infected youth; difficulties in assuring adolescents' participation in research, including clinical trials; and lack of dissemination of effective models for engaging and retaining youth in HIV care and prevention efforts.

In this section, issues related to the care of adolescents are discussed. In addition, more specific recommendations for adolescent HIV care are integrated throughout the guideline. For the purpose of this guideline, adolescents are defined as young persons 13 to 21 years of age. Drugs described in this guideline, and dosages specific to adolescents, are detailed in Appendix B.

Prevention

The teenage years are the usual time that risk-related sexual and drug practices may begin. In a national survey of high school students' sexual behavior, 61 percent of male students and 48 percent of female students had sexual intercourse by graduation (CDC, 1992g). A 1988 national survey of adolescent males reported that in 17-19 year old males living in urban areas, rates of sexual intercourse increased 15 percent over those reported in 1979 (Sonenstein, Pleck, Ku, 1989).

Encouragingly, condom use by adolescents appears to be increasing; the same 1988 survey reported a doubling of reported condom use from 1979 to 1988 (21% to 58%, respectively). However, rates of condom use are disproportionately low among teenagers who participate in behaviors, such as drug and alcohol use, which put them at higher risk for HIV infection (Sonenstein, Pleck, and Ku, 1989). In terms of consistency of condom use, a random-digit dialing telephone survey in Massachusetts found that only 31 percent of the sexually active respondents reported consistent condom use (Hingson, Strunin, Berlin, and Heeren, 1990). Likewise, "survival sex" (sexual intercourse in exchange for food, shelter, or money) puts some adolescents at increased risk of HIV exposure from infected adults. Sexual abuse in childhood is also a predictor for early age of first intercourse in adolescence, thereby compounding the risk for HIV. Non-injectable but behavior-modifying drugs (such as alcohol and crack cocaine) are associated with risk-taking behavior—in particular, unprotected sexual intercourse (Kunins, Hein, and Futterman, 1993).

Information alone is not sufficient to change behavior in adolescents (Rotherman-Borus, Koopman, Haigner, and Davis, 1991), and risk-reduction messages and strategies need to be age-specific (Holtzman, Mathis, Kann et al., 1992; Jemmott, Jemmott and Fong, 1992). Skill-building programs involving adults taking responsibility for motivating adolescents have shown lasting effects up to 2 years after intervention (Ku, Sonenstein, Pleck, 1992; Rotheram-Borus, Koopman, Haignere, and Davies, 1991). Recent national school-based surveys have demonstrated the effects of AIDS education on reducing risk-related behaviors (Holtzman, Anderson, Kann et al., 1991; Holtzman, Mathis, Kann et al., 1992), including a reduction in the number of sexual partners and increased condom use (Forrest, 1992).

Disclosure and Counseling

Age-specific counseling at the time of HIV testing is the first step in appropriate early care for HIV-infected adolescents. Eleven states have specific laws regarding consent, most allowing minors to be tested without parental consent or knowledge (English, 1992).

Providers should note that adolescents are disproportionately affected by the current mandatory HIV-testing policies in Federal education, training, and service programs (Hein, 1991), putting these adolescents at a serious disadvantage in terms of coping with positive HIV test results. For all adolescents, support at the time of test result notification and on an ongoing basis in the form of a supportive adult (parent, guardian, or other) is preferable. It appears that voluntary confidential or anonymous counseling and HIV-testing programs which assure linkage of adolescents to followup care are most effective for this age group (Kunins, Hein, and Futterman, 1993).

Clinical Assessment and Management

Clinical assessment and care are different for adolescents than for young children or adults (Futterman and Hein, 1992). Few studies of HIV progression have included adolescents; however, studies of adolescents with hemophilia suggest that HIV infection progresses more slowly in adolescents than in young children or adults. History-taking, physical examination, and laboratory assessment of the HIV-infected adolescent all need to be conducted and interpreted within the context of age-specific issues.

An appropriate history should include details of sexual and drug use practices including age of initiation, same and opposite sex experiences, sexual identity, and use of condoms or other barrier methods. Psychosocial assessment should include details of living situation, peer group associations, and school and work activities, as well as an assessment of cognitive development and psychiatric history (with attention to suicidal ideation). These factors have implications for the content of counseling, the ability of the patient to cope with HIV infection, and the ongoing evaluation of neurologic manifestations.

The physical examination and staging of HIV infection should take into account the marked changes in body size and composition and organ function that occur during puberty. When assessing development during adolescence, use of the Sexual Maturity Rating Scale of Tanner and Whitehouse (Tanner, 1962) is a more reliable indicator of pubertal development than is chronological age. The immune system, which is nearly fully developed by late childhood, more closely resembles that of adults than that of young children. Likewise, although few normative data exist for CD4 counts in adolescents, available studies reflect adult values (Tollerud, Ildstad, Brown et al., 1990). Other manifestations of HIV progression may differ; in adults, HIV wasting is defined by weight loss, whereas during puberty (when height and weight should be increasing dramatically), wasting should be characterized as failure to gain weight. Because adolescents have the highest rates of STDs of any age group, a screening pelvic or genital examination and laboratory assessment are indicated even for asymptomatic adolescents who have had sexual intercourse. In addition, the provider should consider that the characteristics of the genital tract in young adolescent females predispose them to other STDs and possibly to HIV infection (Bell and Hein, 1984).

Adolescents 13 through 17 years of age were not originally included in clinical trials for HIV-related treatments in numbers large enough to provide valid information (Futterman and Hein, 1992). In 1992, however, several sites were funded to encourage adolescent participation. Until data from these trials are available, a useful, practical approach to adjustment of doses is to begin with pediatric dose schedules for adolescents who are Tanner stage I or II and with adult doses for adolescents who are Tanner stage IV or V (Tanner, 1962). Tanner stage III youth should be monitored particularly closely, as this is the time of most rapid growth. Pubertal changes in body composition and organ function may affect drug distribution and metabolism, thereby necessitating changes in drug dose and interval of drug administration.

To care adequately for HIV-infected youth, primary care providers must first address the barriers that prevent adolescents from accessing care, including payment, consent, and confidentiality. Providers further must be comfortable and conversant with age-specific issues in history-taking (including review of sexual and drug practices) and special aspects of the physical examination (including Tanner staging) and must be able to offer the appropriate range of laboratory tests, including Pap smears and STD screening tests. Ideally, these services should all be provided at one site as needed. Because there are few such ideal service settings, primary care providers of both HIV-infected children and adults should make these accommodations for youth in order to attract and retain them in care.

Areas for Future Research

Many issues related to caring for HIV-infected adolescents remain unexamined and should be put on an agenda for future research. These issues include:

- Studies of the progression of HIV infection in adolescents.

- Elucidation of normal CD4 counts and percentages in adolescents (both healthy and HIV-infected) by Tanner stage, age, and sex.

- Identification of effective ways of expanding participation of youth in treatment programs and clinical trials and assessing the consent process.

■ Evaluation of the impact of various HIV counseling and testing approaches on adolescents (mandatory vs. voluntary; anonymous vs. confidential), including mental health outcomes and effectiveness in linking youth to followup care.

■ Determination of optimal models for primary care of HIV-infected adolescents (e.g., special HIV and/or AIDS programs for adolescents, special HIV-care programs that incorporate adolescents, and adolescent programs that incorporate HIV-infected individuals).

4 Guideline: Early HIV Infection in Infants and Children

Introduction

This chapter is written for the primary care provider and addresses selected issues in the early identification and management of infants and children with HIV infection. For the purpose of this guideline, adolescents are defined as young persons between the ages of 13 and 21 years (see Chapter 3: Caring for Adolescents with Early HIV Infection), children are 2 to 12 years of age, infants are from 30 days of age to age 2, and newborns are from birth to 30 days of age.

Since the screening of blood products began in 1985, perinatal HIV transmission has accounted for 85 percent of all AIDS cases in children less than 13 years of age (CDC, 1987). The perinatal (mother to newborn) transmission rate in large prospective studies is between 13 and 39 percent (Blanche, Rouzioux, Moscato et al., 1989; European Collaborative Study, 1991; Hutto, Parks, Lai et al., 1991; Italian Multicentre Study, 1988; Ryder, Nsa, Hassig et al., 1989). Reports based on seroprevalence and AIDS mortality data suggest that there are 15,000 to 20,000 HIV-infected infants and children in the United States (House Select Committee, 1992; Oleske, 1987).

Perinatal infection exacts a significant toll early in life, with a larger percentage of patients dying in the first year of life than at any other time (Scott, Hutto, Makuch et al., 1989). By 1989, pediatric AIDS had become the eighth leading cause of death in children 1 to 4 years of age in the United States and the sixth leading cause of death in youths 15 to 24 years of age (Chu, Buehler, Oxtoby, and Kilborne, 1991; National Center for Health Statistics, 1992).

Although approximately 75 percent of infants who are exposed to HIV perinatally are not infected, all perinatally exposed infants will suffer the adverse consequences of being born into a family in which one or more adults is infected with HIV. In addition, pediatric HIV infection occurs disproportionately in impoverished minority populations, groups with limited access to health care (Haiken, Hernandez, Mintz, and Boland, 1990; Oleske, 1987). It is also estimated that by the year 2000, approximately 80,000 children will have lost their mothers to HIV and/or AIDS (Michaels and Levine, 1992).

Routine prospective management of perinatally exposed infants and infected children can be provided by primary care providers (Dehovitz, 1990; Oleske, McSherry, Altman et al., 1992). This includes followup of clinical and immune status and general pediatric care, including immunizations. Early diagnosis of HIV-exposed infants can be complicated, and management of children with HIV infection can be difficult—as is true with any chronic multiorgan systemic condition—and may necessitate consultation between the primary health care provider and a specialist in pediatric HIV care. Such collaborative management in infected infants may significantly improve survival and quality of life. In addition, for the symptomatic child, medical and psychosocial issues can be managed optimally through participation in a family-centered case management system or support network often available in the community and targeted towards persons with HIV infection (Novello and Allen, 1991). The definition of family should be expanded in the case of disenfranchised youth where a community-based agency or peer-partner may provide the only support. Such systems or networks are essential in providing the framework for enhanced medical care and treatment and access to clinical drug trials.

In summary, primary care providers utilizing these guidelines and other resources should be able to identify at-risk infants and HIV-infected children; perform routine counseling and diagnostic tests for HIV infection; monitor clinical and immunologic status; provide general pediatric care, including immunizations; and link families to case management and additional counseling, recognizing the effects of the disease on other family members including siblings. Specific situations such as HIV diagnostic testing in infants and evaluation of HIV-related central nervous system (CNS) symptoms, will require consultation with a pediatric HIV specialist.

The pediatric section of this guideline was driven by three major questions that were addressed by an extensive literature review, resulting in the recommendations that follow. The chapter does not address many of the issues related to pediatric HIV infection, which should be examined by future panels.

Diagnosis of HIV Infection in Infants and Children

Nowhere is the need for early diagnosis of HIV infection more pressing than in perinatally exposed infants and children. In these patients, the interval between infection, development of AIDS, and mortality is compressed (Scott, Hutto, Makuch et al., 1989). At birth, infected infants cannot be differentiated from uninfected infants on the basis of clinical and immunologic parameters. Wherever possible, HIV diagnostic testing of infants and children should be incorporated into the schedule of routine pediatric care and immunizations recommended by the American Academy of Pediatrics' Committee on Infectious Diseases and the CDC's Advisory Committee on Immunization Practices. Laboratory diagnosis of HIV-infected newborns and infants is complex and should be done in consultation with a pediatric HIV specialist. Table 2 summarizes the recommendations discussed below.

Recommendation: All infants born to HIV-infected mothers should be monitored to determine HIV status. (Supported by evidence)

Recommendation: In the HIV-exposed infant under 18 months of age, use of virus culture or polymerase chain reaction (PCR) is the preferred method for diagnosis of HIV infection. If these tests are not available, P24 antigen assays should be utilized for diagnosis. One or more of these HIV-specific tests should be done as soon as possible after 1 month of age and, if negative, should be repeated between 3 and 6 months of age. Infants with negative diagnostic tests at 6 months of age should have an HIV antibody test (ELISA) performed at 15 and 18 months of age to document HIV infection status. (Supported by evidence)

Recommendation: In the child over 18 months of age, testing for antibody to HIV using the standard ELISA test with an approved confirmatory test is sufficient for diagnosis of HIV. (Supported by evidence)

Serologic diagnosis of HIV infection in the infant under age 18 is complicated by passive transfer of maternal antibodies across the placenta. The median time to disappearance of maternal antibody in most studies is about 10 months (European Collaborative Study, 1991), but antibody has been reported to persist for as long as 18 months (European Collaborative Study, 1988; Jendis, Tomasik, Hunziker et al., 1988). Thus, immunoglobulin G (IgG) antibody testing alone cannot be used reliably for diagnosis of HIV infection until after 18 months of age. Criteria for the diagnosis of HIV in the perinatally exposed infant under 18 months of age can be formulated based on literature and practical clinical experience.

CDC has utilized a combination of clinical and laboratory criteria for diagnosis of HIV infection in infants and children (CDC, 1987). Prospective studies of infants born to HIV-infected mothers show that most have clinical or immunologic abnormalities (hypergammaglobulinemia, usually IgG or IgA, or low CD4 counts) by 6 months of age (European Collaborative Study, 1991; Hutto, Parks, Lai et al., 1991; Johnson, Nair, Hines et al., 1989; Monforte, Novati, Galli et al., 1990; Tuset, Elorza, Tuset et al., 1990). Common clinical manifestations and HIV-associated conditions in infants and children are listed in Table 3.

Viral culture remains the standard test for diagnosis of HIV in early infancy. Ideally, all perinatally exposed infants should have an HIV viral culture as soon as possible after 1 month of age and again between 3 and 6 months of age if the initial culture was negative. A positive culture constitutes a presumptive diagnosis and should be

Table 2. Diagnosis of infection in HIV-exposed infants

Age	Test	If test is positive	If test is negative
1 month	HIV culture or PCR[1]	Repeat test to confirm diagnosis of infection	Repeat test at age 3-6 months
3-6 months	HIV culture or PCR[1]	Repeat test to confirm diagnosis of infection	Test with ELISA at age 15 months
15 months	ELISA	Repeat test at age 18 months	Repeat test at age 18 months
18 months or older	ELISA	Child is infected[2]	Child is not infected[3]

[1] If HIV culture and PCR are unavailable, p24 antigen testing may be used after 1 month of age.

[2] Serologic diagnosis of HIV infection requires two sets of confirmed HIV serologic assays (ELISA/Western blot) performed at least 1 month apart after 15 months of age.

[3] Confirmation of seronegativity requires two sets of negative ELISAs after 15 months of age in a child with normal clinical and immunoglobulin evaluation.

Note: This table presents recommendations only for the items reviewed by the HIV Panel.

confirmed by a second culture, PCR, or p24 antigen assay. A negative culture result in an infant less than 18 months of age does not rule out infection. Viral culture is available at most larger centers caring for children with HIV infection. Disadvantages of this test include its cost, limited availability, and the length of time to completion (28 days). The PCR amplifies and detects HIV proviral DNA in peripheral blood mononuclear cells from individuals with HIV infection. If facilities for HIV culture or PCR are not available, samples should be sent to a regional center for testing (locations can be found by calling 1-800-TRIALS-A.)

Tests for detection of p24 core protein (p24 antigen) are readily available from most commercial laboratories but are less sensitive than the other tests and should not be used as the only test for HIV infection in the first month of life. Newer p24 assays may offer improved sensitivity by acid dissociation of immune complexes and may soon impact on diagnostic evaluation (DeRossi, Ades, Mammano et al., 1991; Krivine, Yakudima, LeMay et al., 1990; Laure, Rouzioux,

Veber et al., 1988; Miles, Balden, Magpantay et al, 1993; Rogers, Ou, Rayfield et al., 1989; Rudin, Senn, Berger et al., 1991). These tests can be used singly or in combination to diagnose HIV infection in the majority of infants by 6 months of age (Siena Conference, 1992).

A number of newer tests for early neonatal diagnosis of HIV infection are undergoing evaluation but are not yet available for routine clinical use. These include HIV-specific IgA antibody assays and *in vitro* HIV-antibody production assays (Landesman, Weiblen, Mendez et al., 1991; Lee, Nahmias, Lowery et al., 1989; Martin, Long, and Legg, 1991; Pahwa, Chirmule, Leombruno et al., 1989; Quinn, Kline, Halsey et al., 1991; Weiblen, Lee, Cooper et al., 1990).

A perinatally exposed infant 18 months or older who has a normal clinical examination, normal quantitative immunoglobulin, and a normal CD4 count and has had two consecutive negative ELISA antibody tests is presumed not to be HIV infected. Diagnosis in the infant or child over 18 months of age is usually determined by a positive ELISA test confirmed by a Western blot.

Monitoring of CD4 Cells and Initiation of PCP Prophylaxis and Antiretroviral Therapy

The natural history of HIV infection in infants and children differs from that in adolescents and adults primarily through the more rapid onset of clinical symptoms and progression to death. HIV infection has more adverse effects on the function of the developing immune system than infection acquired after the immune system has matured. The progression of HIV infection in both adults and children usually parallels the degree of immune suppression (Bash, Robb, Ascher et al., 1990; Blanche, Tardieu, Duliege et al., 1990; deMartino, Tovo, Galli et al., 1991; Kovacs, Frederick, Church et al., 1991; Nadal, Hunziker, Schüpbach et al., 1989; Thomas, Lubin, Milberg et al., 1987). Thus, it is just as important in children as it is in adolescents and adults to utilize a marker of immune status, so that antiretroviral therapy to delay progression of disease and provide prophylaxis against life-threatening OIs can be instituted while still effective.

The ability to perform reliable CD4 lymphocyte counts on a small volume (less than 3 ml) of whole blood in infants (Denny, Yogev, Gelman et al., 1992), the prognostic value of this marker of immune function, and the availability of this assay in the United States support the selection of CD4 lymphocyte measurement as the primary routine test for monitoring immune status and risk of disease progression in HIV-infected infants and children. See Table 2 for a summary of the recommendations listed below. Drugs and dosages described in this section are detailed in Appendix B.

Table 3. HIV-associated conditions in pediatric HIV infection

Failure to thrive
Generalized lymphadenopathy
Hepatomegaly
Splenomegaly
Persistent oral candidiasis
Parotitis
Recurrent or chronic diarrhea
Encephalopathy
Lymphoid interstitial pneumonitis (LIP)
Hepatitis
Cardiomyopathy
Nephropathy
Recurrent bacterial infections
Opportunistic infections (recurrent viral infections [herpes simplex, herpes zoster], fungal, parasitic)
Malignancies (lymphoma)

Recommendation: CD4 counts and percentages should be obtained in all infants born to HIV-infected mothers at 1, 3, and 6 months of age and then at 3-month intervals until the HIV status of the child is known. Thereafter, CD4 counts and percentages should be monitored at 3- to 6-month intervals in children proven to be HIV infected. (Expert opinion)

Serial monitoring of CD4 cell counts and percentages is the primary method used to assess immune status, risk of disease progression, and the need for prophylaxis against PCP and must be available to all care settings where HIV-exposed or -infected infants and HIV-infected children receive care. The CD4 lymphocyte count has been accepted as the most appropriate surrogate marker to follow immune status in HIV-infected adults (CDC, 1992b); however, until recently, the application of CD4 counts to predict immunosuppression and progression of HIV disease in infants and young children had been limited by the lack of normative data for CD4 lymphocyte counts based on age.

CD4 lymphocyte counts below 500 cells/μl in children are generally associated with the development of OIs, encephalopathy, common bacterial infections, and a poor prognosis (Becherer, Smiley, Matthews et al., 1990; 1988; European Collaborative Study, 1991; Hutto, Parks, Lai et al., 1991; Italian Multicentre Study, 1988; Johnson, Nair, Hines et al., 1989; Scott, Hutto, Makuch et al., 1989; Smith, Forbes, Cooper et al., 1991; Ujhelyi, Fuchs, Králl et al., 1990).

PCP Prophylaxis_____

Recommendation: Prophylaxis for PCP should be initiated if the CD4 count falls below age-adjusted normal values, if the percentage of CD4 cells is less than or equal to 20 percent, or after an episode of PCP regardless of CD4 count. In the infant born to an HIV-infected mother, PCP prophylaxis should be started if any of the age-adjusted CD4 criteria are met, even if the child's HIV infection status is not confirmed (see Table 2). The drug of choice for prophylaxis is TMP-SMX. (Suggested by evidence)

PCP is the most frequent OI in children less than 1 year of age who have HIV infection. It carries a high fatality rate, almost 40 percent, even with intravenous TMP-SMX or pentamidine treatment and has a poor prognosis for long-term survival (Bernstein, Bye, and Rubinstein, 1989; Kovacs, Frederick, Church et al., 1991; Oxtoby, 1990; Vernon, Holzman, Lewis et al., 1988). It is likely that the diagnosis of HIV infection and initiation of PCP prophylaxis where appropriate will improve overall outcomes in HIV-infected infants, children, or adolescents.

The observation that PCP could occur in infants under 1 year of age with absolute CD4 lymphocyte counts above 200 cells/μl but usually below 1500 cells/μl suggests that infants have higher normal levels of CD4 lymphocytes than adults, as well as indicating that 1500 cells/μl is a reasonable count for initiation of PCP prophylaxis for the infant under the age of 1 year (CDC, 1991a; Connor, Bagarazzi, McSherry et al., 1991; Frederick, Mascola, Evans et al., 1989; Kovacs, Frederick, Church et al., 1991; Leibovitz, Rigaud, Pollack et al., 1990; Rutstein, 1991). Age-adjusted CD4 data for normal pediatric populations supports this observation (Denny, Yogev, Gelman et al., 1992). Algorithm 7 (Appendix A) details these age-adjusted data (CDC, 1991a). Abnormal CD4 counts should be confirmed, but PCP prophylaxis should be initiated pending results of these confirmatory studies.

Studies in progress may suggest that PCP prophylaxis should be initiated in at-risk and infected infants 1 month to 1 year of age, regardless of CD4 count or percentage. The provider should review the literature often for new developments.

Experience with children with cancer undergoing immunosuppressive chemotherapy showed that PCP can be prevented with chemoprophylaxis (Hughes, Kuhn, Chaudhary et al., 1977). Studies of PCP prophylaxis in HIV-exposed or -infected infants are not available. TMP-SMX is the drug of choice for PCP prophylaxis in infants and children over 1 month of age (see Appendix B-1). Alternative prophylactic regimens have not been the focus of this guideline, but such recommendations have been published by the Public Health Service (CDC, 1991a).

87

Antiretroviral Therapy_____

Recommendation: Antiretroviral therapy should be initiated for (a) all infants and children with symptomatic HIV infection (suggested by evidence); (b) in any HIV-infected infant or child whose CD4 count falls below the following age-adjusted thresholds: <1750 cells/μl for infants birth to 12 months, <1000 cells/μl for infants 13 to 24 months, <750 cells/μl for children 2 to 6 years, and <500 cells/μl for children over 6 years of age; (c) in any HIV-infected infant less than 1 year of age with a CD4 count <30 percent; between 1 and 2 years with a CD4 count <25 percent; and (d) for all other ages through adolescence, a CD4 count <20 percent (see Algorithm 7, Appendix A) (expert opinion).

The limited number of specific antiretroviral agents available today and the past delay in the initiation of controlled studies in children have resulted in a limited literature on which to base recommendations regarding initiation of antiretroviral therapy in children and adolescents less than 18 years of age. There are no data on early use of antiretroviral agents in asymptomatic infants, children, or adolescents. It seems reasonable to expect that early initiation of treatment of HIV infection should be more effective than waiting for symptomatic disease to develop (see Table 3), with its attendant greater viral burden. However, risks and benefits of early therapy should be discussed with the parent, guardian, and child (depending on age), and a mutual decision should be made. As more antiretroviral agents become available, the concern regarding development of drug resistance becomes less of a reason for withholding ZDV in earlier stages of the infection (Krasinski, 1991; McKinney, 1991; Pizzo, 1990).

Children with AIDS-defining illness should be treated with antiretroviral therapy; see Appendix B-2 for dosing information. Other infants and children who have symptomatic disease (see Table 3), with the possible exception of isolated lymphadenopathy or hepatomegaly, should also receive antiretroviral therapy.

The use of CD4 lymphocyte counts to predict which asymptomatic children should be placed on antiretroviral therapy is not established by the available literature. None of the protocols to date have used CD4 counts alone as an inclusion or exclusion criterion for enrollment in clinical trials. From a study of 88 HIV-infected children with advanced disease (McKinney, Maha, Connor et al., 1991) and a similar clinical trial of 35 children with less symptomatic disease (McKinney, Pizzo, Scott et al., 1990), it can be inferred that children with CD4 counts below 500 cells/μl are candidates for antiretroviral therapy. In the latter study, those children with CD4 counts below 500 cells/μl at entry into the trial had less increase in CD4 counts during antiretroviral therapy than those with CD4 counts greater than 500 cells/μl at study enrollment. Thus, guidelines were developed using age-related CD4 counts for initiating antiretroviral therapy in infants and children (National Pediatric HIV Resource Center, 1993). Antiretroviral therapy should be used only in those children with proven HIV infection and after the uncertainties of therapy are discussed with the parent or guardian and child (see Diagnosis of HIV Infection in Infants and Children in this chapter).

ZDV and ddI are currently the only antiretroviral agents approved by the FDA for treatment of HIV infection in children under age 13. ZDV is currently the drug of choice for initial therapy in HIV-infected children as outlined above. In clinical trials, children treated with ZDV have demonstrated improvement in weight gain and cognitive functions. They have also shown a stabilization in CD4 lymphocyte counts, a reduction in serum and CSF p24 antigen levels, and a decrease in immunoglobulin levels (Blanche, Caniglia, Fischer et al., 1988; Gupta, Ravipati, Slade et al., 1989; Knutsen, Bouhasin, Gioia, and Mueller, 1989; Pizzo, Eddy, Falloon et al., 1988).

Appendix B-2 describes common side effects of antiretroviral therapy. The most frequent side effects of ZDV include anemia and neutropenia. Approximately 25 percent of children receiving ZDV require dose reduction because of these side effects, but toxicity requiring drug discontinuation occurs very rarely. Other side effects include insomnia, vomiting, neuropathy/myopathy, headaches, and hyperactivity; these are most commonly seen in the first few weeks of therapy and rarely require dose alteration or drug discontinuation. Because of the above toxicities, a complete blood count, liver function, and creatine phosphokinase should be monitored regularly (Blanche, Caniglia, Fischer et al., 1988; McKinney, Pizzo, Scott et al., 1990; Pizzo, Eddy, Falloon et al., 1988).

ddI is approved for use in symptomatic adult and pediatric patients who are not adequately responding to, are intolerant to, or have a contraindication to ZDV. Therapeutic decisions to change from ZDV to another antiretroviral medication in HIV-infected children should be done in consultation with a specialist. Treatment with ddI has been associated with improvement in both clinical and laboratory parameters. In contrast to ZDV, ddI is not usually associated with hematologic toxicity; rather, its principal toxicities are pancreatitis and peripheral neuropathy. Peripheral retinal atrophy was observed in a few children treated with ddI, but its clinical significance is unknown (Butler, Husson, Balis et al., 1991).

ddC (zalcitabine) is one of the more potent agents against HIV *in vitro* but has less penetration of the CNS than other nucleosides. The dose-limiting toxicity for ddC is peripheral neuropathy, whereas rash and aphthous stomatitis are less severe side effects. Data are available on only a few children treated with ddC, and improvements in some markers have been noted (Pizzo, Butler, Balis et al., 1989). Currently, a trial of ddC therapy in children who have had disease progression while on ZDV is ongoing, and a trial of combination therapy with ZDV is underway.

Although the long-term adverse effects of antiretroviral agents are unknown, their beneficial effects in infants and children support their use.

Neurologic Testing in Infants and Children

HIV infection in infants, children, and adolescents results in a wide spectrum and high incidence of neurologic diseases (Belman, Ultmann, Horoupian et al., 1985; Brouwers, Belman, and Epstein, 1991; Epstein, Sharer, Oleske et al., 1986; Mintz, 1992; Mintz and Epstein, 1992; Sharer, Epstein, Cho et al., 1986; Sharer and Mintz, in press; Shaw, Hahn, Epstein et al., 1985). Progressive neurologic disease in HIV-infected infants and children has been reported to occur at an incidence ranging from 9 to 19 percent in prospective studies conducted in Europe (European Collaborative Study, 1988, 1990; Laverda, Cogo, Condini et al., 1990). Retrospective studies conducted in the United States in older HIV-infected children uncovered an incidence of 75 to 90 percent for neurodevelopmental delays or regression and neuropsychological deficits (Belman, Ultmann, Horoupian et al., 1985; Mintz, 1992). The true incidence of HIV-related CNS disease in HIV-infected children is not yet clear and awaits completion of prospective studies.

Early onset of an HIV-associated progressive encephalopathy has most commonly been noted in infants and children with symptomatic HIV disease. In children with perinatal HIV infection, the clinical signs of neurologic dysfunction may appear as early as 2 months of age and as late as 5 years or longer after birth (Mintz, Epstein, and Koenigsberger, 1989). Longitudinal and retrospective studies suggest that, after a period of normal development, three neurodevelopmental courses may occur: rapid progression; steady, subacute progression; or stepwise decline with relatively stable periods (Belman, Ultmann, Horoupian et al., 1985; Epstein, Sharer, Oleske et al., 1986; Mintz, Epstein, and Koenigsberger, 1989).

HIV may cause neurologic dysfunction through the direct or indirect effects of a primary infection of the brain with HIV (Epstein, Goudsmit, Paul et al., 1989; Epstein, Sharer, Oleske et al., 1986; Fauci, 1988; Heyes, Robinow, Lane, and Markey, 1989; Michaels, Price, and Rosenblum, 1988; Mintz, Rapaport, Oleske et al., 1989; Odeh, 1990; Price, Brew, Sidtis et al., 1988; Shaw, Hahn, Epstein et al., 1985).

Algorithm 8 (Appendix A) summarizes the following recommendations.

Recommendation: A neurologic examination, including an age-related developmental assessment, should be performed on all HIV-exposed infants and HIV-infected infants and children at the initial assessment. A neurologic examination should be performed at each clinical visit and an age-related developmental assessment should be done every 3 months for the first 24 months of life and every 6 months thereafter. (Expert opinion)

The most frequent CNS manifestations in infants and children with HIV infection include: (1) impaired brain growth; (2) motor dysfunction and, in older children, attention and memory difficulties; (3) loss or plateau of previously acquired milestones; and (4) cognitive impairment (Belman, 1990; Belman, Ultmann, Horoupian et al., 1985; Byers, 1989; Haney, Yale-Loehr, Nussbaum, and Gellad, 1989; Laverda, Cogo, Condini et al., 1990; Mintz, 1992; Mintz, Epstein, and Koenigsberger, 1989; Price, Inglese, Jacobs et al., 1988; Rosenblum, Levy, and Bredesen, 1988). Neurologic evaluation of the HIV-infected infant, child, or adolescent should include a complete history, as well as physical and neurologic examinations and an age-related developmental assessment (Mintz, 1992).

HIV-infected children with developmental delay and other neurologic deficits should be evaluated by a specialist to assess the type, extent, or stage of developmental disability (Crocker, 1989). These assessments will provide primary care physicians, parents, counselors, psychologists, educators, and physical, occupational, and speech therapists with information that will help them to design and manage intervention programs on an individual basis (Crocker, 1989; Haiken, Hernandez, Mintz, and Boland, 1991; Mintz, 1992; Mintz and Epstein, 1992). Although the value of early intervention programs has not been established, under a program tailored for the HIV-infected child, it is anticipated that quality of life will be improved (Mintz, 1992).

Recommendation: Baseline computerized tomographic (CT) scans or magnetic resonance imaging (MRI) is recommended at the time of diagnosis of HIV infection in infants and children. Subsequently, if CNS symptoms occur, neuroimaging studies, should be repeated and CSF obtained for analysis. Serial MRIs and CT scans are not indicated for the routine care of HIV-infected infants and children in the absence of CNS symptoms. (Expert opinion)

A baseline CT scan or MRI of the brain is recommended, where possible, in HIV-infected infants and children as an indication for initiation of antiretroviral treatments in those noted to have abnormal studies and to provide a comparison for subsequent neuroimaging studies when clinical evidence of focal pathology, obstructive lesions, atypical CNS manifestations, or evidence of progressive neurologic disease occurs. CT examinations of the brain may show variable degrees of loss of cerebral parenchymal volume, white matter changes, or calcification of the basal ganglia or frontal periventricular white matter (Belman, 1990; Belman, Ultmann, Horoupian et al., 1985; Haney, Yale-Loehr, Nussbaum, and Gellad, 1989; Price, Inglese, Jacobs et al., 1988). Serial CT scans may incur substantial cost, yet yield little clinical benefit. A report of serial MRI examinations did not influence intervention strategies or clinical outcome and, although they are more sensitive than CT scans, also cannot be recommended for routine use at this time (Chamberlain, Nichols, and Chase, 1991; Mintz, 1992).

CSF examination — when obtained for an evaluation of abnormal CNS findings — should include, in addition to routine studies, bacterial, fungal, and viral cultures. OIs of the CNS in HIV-infected children include *M. tuberculosis,* cryptococcosis, toxoplasmosis, herpes simplex, JC virus, and cytomegalovirus. OIs of the CNS in infants and young children are relatively uncommon compared with older children, adolescents, and adults (Belman, 1990; Mintz, 1992; Mintz and Epstein, 1992; Mintz, Epstein, and Koenigsberger, 1989).

The differential diagnosis of CNS symptoms in the HIV-infected infant or child includes neoplasms (especially primary CNS lymphomas), OIs, HIV primary encephalopathy, and CNS bleeding (Belman, 1990; Epstein, DiCarlo, Joshi et al., 1988; Haney, Yale-Loehr, Nussbaum, and Gellad, 1989). Intracerebral hemorrhage occurs most commonly in the setting of immune thrombocytopenia or in conjunction with infection (Epstein, Sharer, Oleske et al., 1986; Park, Belman, Kim et al., 1990).

HIV-associated neuropathies and myopathies, although common in adults, have been reported rarely in young children and infants (Dalakas and Pezeshkpour, 1988; Mintz, 1992; Mintz and Epstein, 1992; Parry, 1988; Simpson, 1992). However, these disorders can occur as an adverse effect of antiretroviral therapy (Walter, Drucker, McKinney, and Wilfert, 1991). Spinal cord syndromes can also occur in the HIV-infected child (Dickson, Belman, and Kim, 1989; Mintz, 1992; Mintz and Epstein, 1992; Sharer, Dowling, Michaels et al., 1990; Sharer and Mintz, in press).

Recommendation: After exclusion of other diagnoses, infants and children who have primary HIV CNS disease should be treated with antiretroviral therapy and referred to a pediatric neurologist with expertise in HIV infection, if available, or a specialist in HIV care. (Suggested by evidence) Support and rehabilitation services, such as nutritional supplementation, physical, occupational, or speech

therapy, and early intervention programs, should be considered as part of the comprehensive management of HIV-infected infants and children with CNS involvement. (Expert opinion)

Brain growth and cognitive deficits in children with HIV-associated encephalopathy were shown to improve after 6 months of continuous infusion of ZDV therapy (Brouwers, Moss, Wolters et al., 1990; DeCarli, Fugate, Falloon et al., 1991). However, some children, after initial improvement, may experience a neurologic deterioration on long-term ZDV therapy (Mintz, 1992; Mintz and Epstein, 1992; Tudor-Williams, St. Clair, McKinney et al., 1992). Although alternative antiretrovirals may be useful in helping such children (Butler, Husson, Balis et al., 1991; Wolters, Brouwers, and Moss, 1990), multicenter trials examining this question have yet to be completed.

Advanced neurologic disease may affect functions, such as swallowing, which can lead to poor nutritional status (Mintz, 1992). In such circumstances, use of either nasogastric or gastrostomy feeding tubes may become necessary. Further deterioration in nutritional status despite nutritional supplementation with tube feeding may necessitate institution of total parenteral alimentation (Mintz and Epstein, 1992).

Areas for Future Research

The panel identified the following areas for future research:

■ Routine HIV testing of newborns.

■ Supportive care and its impact on quality of life.

■ School attendance and special education needs.

■ The need for subspecialty care, including dental care.

■ The impact of limited access to and availability of health care for the impoverished families that are disproportionately affected by HIV-infection.

■ Use of intravenous immunoglobulins and other modalities for the prophylaxis of infections other than PCP and recurrent bacterial infection.

5 Guideline: Case Management for Persons Living with HIV

Introduction

The primary care provider should coordinate the care plan of an individual with HIV in the early stages of infection. As infection progresses, however, the patient, family, significant other, and provider may require a more comprehensive case management system, depending on need and the availability of services in the community. Patients, and their families and significant others, ultimately determine their need for case management services.

Case management is a patient-centered process which has been used to augment and coordinate existing care systems. Its goals are to access health and mental health care for patients; provide or obtain social support services; and empower patients, family members, and significant others. The means of achieving these goals include providing education; creating connections between careseekers and caregivers; promoting active participation of the patient, family, and significant others in developing care plans; and acknowledging and complementing the important support given by family and significant others.

Objectives common to most case management systems are to:

- Assist patients, family, and significant others in achieving a coordinated set of services with client advocacy as an emphasis.

- Provide counseling on diagnosis and its implications, education about prevention and treatment, and necessary health care.

- Complete psychosocial assessments and integrate these with medical and nursing assessments.

- Develop achievable care plans, integrating psychosocial and health care goals.

- Link patients to one or more needed services.

- Support the patient with followthrough and continuation of services.

- Monitor and track patients to determine use, availability, and appropriateness of services.

- Reassess, together with the patient, family, and significant other, the plan and goals if the original plan is not working or cannot be achieved.

- Maintain records of unmet needs to be used in planning and advocacy efforts.

- Maintain records on each patient for evaluation of case management services.

The psychosocial complications of HIV infection may create difficulties as serious as those caused by medical and physical problems. In fact, most individuals coping and living with HIV infection require some level of assistance with financial, legal, emotional, and social support systems at some stage of their infections (Martin, 1990). Contemporary health care systems and social services are not well designed for providing such psychological and social support (Shulman and Mantell, 1988).

Case management is not a panacea for the shortcomings in the health care or social services systems. It is a method for coordinating the provision of services within a community to effect more positive and sustained health outcomes. It cannot, of itself, develop needed resources, nor can it unilaterally manage cases. As is the case with other services for HIV-infected individuals, there are significant regional differences in availability of funding for case management. In some communities, essentially no resources exist to develop or implement case management services; in others, case management services may exist but may not be coordinated, resulting in duplication of services (Moore, 1992).

The recommendations in this guideline are intended to assist primary care providers and persons with HIV to define their case management needs and to utilize existing case management systems. Most of the recommendations are based on published literature, and others are based on panel consensus.

Types of Case Management Services

There is no single model for a case management system. Case management services can be delivered in several settings: primary care sites (physicians' offices, community health clinics, preventive nursing services), secondary care facilities (community or general hospitals), or tertiary care settings (specialty hospitals and rehabilitation facilities), as well as within community-based organizations or through local and State public agencies. Case management systems can be local or regional and can be adapted to urban settings or rural areas (Andrews, Preston, Howell, and Keyes, 1989; Benjamin, Lee, and Solkowitz, 1988; Jellinek, 1988; Rounds, 1988; Schott, 1988; Sierra Health Foundation, 1992). They may range from single-focus, coordinating services by an independent provider to complex, integrated regional networks of providers and services.

Access to Case Management Services

Recommendation: All primary care providers should be knowledge-able about the uses of case management and should develop referral mechanisms to case management services in their community. Methods for accomplishing this include: continuing education and training, contracting with a local or regional case management system, or employing a case manager to assist in the primary care setting. (Expert opinion)

Case management has become a prominent coordinating mechanism for HIV patient care. Although case management's clinical effectiveness and cost efficiency have yet to be rigorously examined (Harder and Kibbe, 1991; Kemper, 1988), it appears to be a valid coordinating system on a conceptual level (Blomberg and Flynn, 1989; Jellinek, 1988). There is literature that supports the utility of case management as a coordinating system in the fields of mental illness (Kane, 1985), developmental disabilities (Harris and Bergman, 1987; Honnard, 1985), and gerontology (Benjamin, 1988; Capitman, Haskins, and Bernstein, 1986; Emlet, 1982). More specific to HIV infection, case management has been shown to be critical in the care of infected injection drug users (Nix and Cabaj, 1992; Pincus-Strom, 1989), women with children, and children in foster care settings (Robert Wood Johnson Foundation, 1991).

The literature and professional consensus suggest that there is no single structure for case management, but rather that a number of systems are evolving which include pragmatic mixtures of features unique to geographic areas, settings, and populations served (Kane, 1985; Wilson and Coover, 1985). Two models of case management predominate in the care of HIV-infected individuals. The choice of model is often based on the severity of the patient's illness. In the early stages of HIV infection, case management is usually driven by the need for community-based services, such as housing and concerns regarding confidentiality and job security. At this stage, case management is usually performed by a social worker. In the later, more severe stages of HIV infection, medical care service needs become paramount, and case management is typically performed by a nurse. For the individual patient, there needs to be coordination and continuity as the transition occurs from a community-based to a medical-based case management system (Indyk and Wade, 1992; Mor, Piette, and Fleishman, 1989).

Process of Case Management

Recommendation: Case management should include intake, assessment of patient needs, and development, implementation, and monitoring of a case management plan with periodic assessments. (Expert opinion)

Piette, Fleishman, Mor, and Thompson (1992) outline steps for case management plans which include:

1. Intake and screening: identification of those requiring, seeking, or eligible for a particular service.

2. Assessment of patient needs: a comprehensive evaluation to determine the patient's situation and his or her strengths and weaknesses. This may be completed by one individual or may be the result of a team process with various persons (staff, patient, family, significant other, health care providers, or other agencies) contributing data and perceptions that will help formulate the case management plan.

3. Development of a written care plan: the setting of goals and objectives, and agreement on the strategically sequenced actions to be taken by each team member in meeting those health care, psychosocial, and/or community goals.

4. Implementation of the plan: translation of the plan into practice through referral, coordination, counseling, advocacy, and task activities to reach the pre-established goals. This often involves skills development and supportive counseling to empower the patient and family to take the greatest possible control of the plan.

5. Monitoring: activities designed to assure that needed services are being provided, verify that the case plan is being executed effectively, and determine to what extent progress is being made.

6. Reassessment: a periodic reevaluation conducted within an established time frame or as needs or circumstances change.

7. Updating: repeat steps 2 to 6, as necessary.

8. Disposition and termination: agreed-upon criteria for concluding the case manager-patient relationship. These criteria may include attainment of goals, geographic relocation, patient dissatisfaction with the service, or death. Case management services are frequently extended after the death of the patient to assist the family or significant others in the grieving process and to assure that arrangements for child care are successfully completed.

Recommendation: Case management should be formalized by a comprehensive written care plan, with objectives carefully delineated as to types of services required, responsible party (provider, agency, patient, family, or case manager), and specific time frame. Patients or parents/guardians should be able to select those specific services they require at a given point in time. (Expert opinion)

The literature suggests that the range of services which are responsive to identified needs of patients and their families or significant others should be made available (Martin, 1990; Mor, Piette, and Fleishman, 1989). These services may include: legal, housing, spiritual, and education/recreational services; entitlement and employment assistance; financial planning; counseling; transportation; vocational rehabilitation; developmental assessment and early intervention for children; medical, nursing, and home health care; pharmaceutical services; drug-dependency treatment; HIV prevention; advocacy; and long-term and hospice care.

The location and resources of the primary care provider, as well as the patient's personal resources and those available in the community, will influence the nature of a specific case management plan and the ability to provide needed services appropriately and effectively. In addition, the nature and degree of defined responsibility for actions and advocacy need to be delineated clearly among the participants in case management (e.g., the case manager, the patient, the family, and significant others) (Benjamin, Lee, and Solkowitz, 1988).

Case managers should recognize that plans may need to be revised to address unplanned changes in the patient's circumstances or in the external service systems.

Case Management Personnel

Recommendation: Case management programs should be directed by individuals knowledgeable about both the clinical nature of HIV and issues affecting service delivery. The qualifications for a case manager may vary, but at a minimum, case managers should have: (a) a working knowledge of their clients' HIV disease process based on medical and nursing assessments; (b) knowledge of and contact with services in immediate and neighboring communities, health care and social services agencies, and public entitlement programs; (c) resourcefulness and creativity in accessing required services; and (d) interpersonal skills which allow effective interaction with clients and multiple providers in households, communities, and medical settings while maintaining a spirit of hope and empathy. (Expert opinion)

In HIV service programs, case managers rarely represent a single discipline. A variety of providers, including social workers, nurses, physicians, psychologists, case management assistants, technical support staff, peer counselors, and volunteers, can be utilized effectively with specific job descriptions and functions to provide the needed level of services in a timely fashion. The literature suggests that, because of the complex interaction between medical and psychosocial issues in HIV infection, case management programs should be directed and supervised by professional level staff and utilize a range of other paid and volunteer staff as patient needs dictate (Blomberg and Flynn, 1989; Hazard, Shervington, Stroud et al., 1989; Sonsel, Paradise, and Stroup, 1988).

Areas for Future Research

The panel recommends the following areas for future research:

- Evaluation of cost and efficiency of various case management models.

- Evaluation and comparison of the role of foster families, extended families, and group homes in the care of HIV-infected children.

- Evaluation of optimal timing of initiation of case management programs.

6 Issues and Challenges: Access to and Availability of Care

Introduction

Individuals infected with HIV will require a broad array of services throughout the course of their infection. Thus, providers need to be aware of and concerned about the availability of services and patients' access to such services. This chapter familiarizes the provider with issues affecting access to and availability of care and provides guidance in anticipating and overcoming barriers to providing and accessing care.

Problems in Health Care Coverage for Early Intervention Services

It is estimated that in 1990 nearly 36 million Americans, or 16.6 percent of the Nation's nonelderly population, were without health insurance (Employee Benefit Research Institute, 1992). The problem appears to be significantly greater for the HIV-infected population. Nearly 30 percent of persons with AIDS lack any form of health care coverage (Andrulis, Weslowski, and Gage, 1989; Harmon, 1992). At primary health care facilities funded under the Ryan White CARE Act, more than 40 percent of the patients are reported to be uninsured (Andrulis, Weslowski, and Gage, 1989).

Private Coverage and the HIV-Infected Population_____

About two-thirds of Americans have private insurance, mostly through employment-based policies (Employee Benefit Research Institute, 1992). It is estimated, however, that less than 30 percent of persons with AIDS who are hospitalized are privately insured, indicating that a significant portion of the HIV-infected population has encountered problems in obtaining or maintaining private health insurance coverage (Andrulis, Weslowski, and Gage, 1989).

Reasons for limited private sector coverage of HIV-infected persons include the shift in the demographics of the epidemic to disadvantaged populations who traditionally have lacked access to employment-based private health insurance (Caplan, 1990). In addition, some insurers have sought to minimize their exposure to the cost of HIV infection in a variety of ways including increasing the use of medical underwriting, which seeks to identify and often exclude individuals considered to be at risk of incurring high medical expenses. Practices such as asking about applicants' sexual orientation, assuming an association between certain occupations and sexual preference, and refusing to sell insurance in certain geographic areas believed to have a high prevalence of individuals at risk for HIV infection, such as gay men, are examples of minimizing insurance risk. In addition, persons covered before the HIV infection was recognized can face potential cancellation of personal coverage, exorbitant increases in premiums, job immobility due to fear of not qualifying for insurance coverage at a new place of employment, or annual caps on expenditures for certain services, such as prescription drugs.

To address the range of problems identified above, a number of States have enacted a variety of policies and programs. Although these State efforts are likely to improve the ability of many HIV-infected persons to obtain and maintain private insurance coverage, they suffer from fragmentation of efforts and restrictions on the States' regulatory purview.

Public-Sector Coverage for HIV-Infected Individuals___

For HIV-infected persons who have lost or cannot obtain private health care coverage, two publicly supported health care financing programs, Medicare and Medicaid, potentially provide financial access to needed health care. Although best known for the protection it provides to the elderly, Medicare also provides health care coverage to certain disabled persons. However, the program's focus on these two populations, combined with its long eligibility waiting periods, make its protection minimal for persons with early HIV infection.

The Federal-State Medicaid program offers greater protection to persons with more advanced HIV infection. However, although the percentage of persons in the early stages of HIV infection who are covered by or eligible for Medicaid is not known, an estimated 40 percent of all persons with AIDS are covered by Medicaid at some point in their illness (Congressional Research Service, 1988).

In general, Medicaid is available to two groups of low-income persons: (a) individuals who are aged, blind, or disabled and (b) pregnant women, children, or members of families with dependent children. In the early stages of the HIV epidemic, most persons who were aware of their HIV infection had advanced disease and so were able to obtain Medicaid coverage through a disability determination. However, in the early and often asymptomatic stages of HIV infection, it has been difficult to meet the definition of disability. Medicaid coverage is therefore generally not available to persons with early HIV infection, unless they qualify as a pregnant woman, a child, or as a member of a family with dependent children.

The program's income eligibility standards vary widely across individual States as well as across the three groups identified above. Even for those HIV-infected persons who gain Medicaid eligibility, there is great variability in Medicaid program policies across States. Although Medicaid programs offer a benefit package that often includes more services than many private insurance plans, some States have imposed significant limits on the number of units of services that will be covered under the program. In addition, despite the fact that primary care physicians may need to spend significantly more time with HIV-infected patients, in many States these physicians may only be reimbursed by Medicaid for less than half of what they would have received under either Medicare or private insurance. This may discourage physicians from caring for individuals with HIV (Physician Payment Review Commission, 1993).

Recognizing that the problems created by low Medicaid reimbursement rates are often quite significant, a number of States have undertaken initiatives designed to increase access to primary and preventive care for certain priority populations. For example, some States have increased Medicaid reimbursement rates to providers for a variety of HIV-related primary care activities, elected to cover case management services under their Medicaid programs, or obtained Federal waivers to expand the scope of community-based services covered under their Medicaid programs. Primary care providers can obtain information about their States' Medicaid initiatives by calling the State HIV hot lines listed in Appendix C.

In addition to Medicaid, a number of other public programs assist HIV-infected persons. For example, the Ryan White CARE Act authorizes States to use a portion of their funds to purchase health insurance continuation coverage and to support a drug-reimbursement program for HIV-infected individuals. However, available resources are often insufficient to meet the demands of these drug reimbursement programs.

Availability of Early Intervention Services and Providers

Similar to the health care financing system, the health care delivery system needs to be better equipped to meet the multiple requirements of HIV-infected persons. These requirements can best be met by developing coordinated and continuous systems of care for HIV-infected individuals and increasing the availability of health care services for this population.

Coordination of Available Services_____

Because of the fragmentation of the current system of care, persons with early HIV infection may encounter significant obstacles in obtaining comprehensive, coordinated care. Providers attempting to function within a delivery system that is not able to address the multiple needs of their patients encounter difficulty finding others who will accept referrals and experience the effects of inadequate support resources.

Throughout the United States, efforts are underway at both the State and local levels to design systems of care that provide services, including early intervention services, to HIV-infected individuals in a more coordinated and efficient manner (Auerbach, 1992; Merzel, Crystal, Sambamoorthi et al., 1992; National Commission on AIDS, 1991). Although no single care delivery model is appropriate for all communities, an essential component of many of the coordinated care systems being developed is that of case management. (For a further discussion of case management, see Chapter 5.)

The cost of developing and operating coordinated care activities is substantial. Funding for many of these efforts comes from the government (Intergovernmental Health Policy Project, 1991). However, as in many other areas related to the HIV epidemic, current public funding is not sufficient to address the needs of communities throughout the United States. The panel supports the need for additional funding for the development of delivery systems which would enable providers to effectively address the needs of HIV-infected persons in a coordinated, cost-effective, and compassionate manner.

Availability of Services_____

The multiple needs of the HIV-infected population require a wide range of skilled personnel, including: physicians, nurses, physician assistants, dentists, eye doctors, psychologists, social workers, counselors, case managers, home health care workers, nutritionists, pharmacists, and patient advocates. With increasing numbers of HIV-infected patients, however, these providers are severely constrained by limited capacity and resources. The pressures of caring for larger numbers of patients are felt also by health care institutions. In most communities, a small number of clinics and hospitals care for a disproportionate number of patients with HIV infection, in part because of their location, in part because of reimbursement issues, and in part because of the reluctance of some health care providers to treat HIV-infected or AIDS patients (Intergovernmental Health Policy Project, 1990).

Even under ideal circumstances, it is difficult to develop a professional staff willing and committed to caring for HIV-infected patients. Provider reluctance to care for HIV-infected individuals has varied and complex roots. Physicians, nurses, and other health care providers may lack familiarity with and understanding of treatment for HIV infection, fear becoming infected, be uncomfortable in treating gay men or injection drug users, and be unprepared to work with severely ill or dying young patients who have multiple physical and psychological needs. Providers also may be discouraged from treating patients with HIV infection by a combination of limited financial incentives and the increased time required for treating these patients. Although there have been many providers dedicated to HIV care for the past decade, some providers do not perceive an ethical obligation to care for patients with HIV infection.

Increasing Access to and Availability of Services

The panel believes that comprehensive health care coverage is required to ensure access to quality health care services. In addition, increasing the number of providers willing to care for HIV-infected individuals is central to increasing and improving early intervention services. Until these ultimate goals are reached, however, the panel suggests the following strategies:

- Eliminating insurance restrictions on those at risk for HIV infection or who are HIV-infected.

- Enabling HIV-infected individuals to obtain self-insurance, e.g., by establishing statewide insurance pools for persons who would otherwise not be able to obtain third-party private coverage because of preexisting medical problems.

- Enabling Medicaid to cover all low-income people with HIV infection.

- Increasing Medicaid reimbursement rates.

- Allowing infected individuals who are disabled to enroll in Medicare during the 2-year waiting period.

- Funding the Ryan White CARE Act to meet the needs of HIV-infected individuals by reflecting actual costs.

- Enhancing access to potentially lifesaving HIV-related drugs.

- Promoting financial coverage of early intervention services.

- Addressing underlying attitudes of all members of society.

- Focusing on attitudes of the full range of caregivers through intensive education and training.

- Supporting and recognizing providers who care for HIV-infected persons.

- Recruiting providers to care for HIV-infected persons through development of innovative programs such as an "HIV corps" of providers or special incentive programs.

The following strategies may be used by providers and patients to optimize access to and availability of care:

- Become familiar with broad issues in health care access, particularly with potential obstacles to accessing care.

- Discuss these issues with patients in the context of their HIV care requirements and the limitations of their specific health care coverage.

- Employ a case-management approach to care planning which anticipates future health care needs of individuals alongside the realities of their coverage, links patients to medical and social services, advocates for patients, assists them in accessing care, avoids duplication of services, and ensures cohesive, coordinated, and comprehensive care (see Chapter 5 for a discussion of case management).

- Organize and participate in community programs that support and recognize providers of early HIV care while promoting access and availability of services for HIV-infected individuals.

The HIV epidemic compels providers to acquire new information and skills and public and private policymakers to develop new systems to meet challenges. Although progress has been made and individual providers and programs can take pride in their accomplishments, the overall response from our health care delivery system has not, at present, met all of the existing needs for HIV-related health services (National Commission on AIDS, 1993).

As the number of HIV-infected persons continues to increase, the need for care and providers also increases. The changing geographic distribution of the disease, with HIV infection no longer concentrated in only a handful of cities but spread across the country, will place increasing demands on delivery sites and providers formerly unaffected by the epidemic. This guideline is an important step towards reducing barriers to care caused by a lack of medical knowledge, but significant additional steps need to be taken if the promises of early intervention are to become realities. Both public- and private-sector efforts must be directed toward the development of more effective and compassionate delivery systems that will be able to implement the recommendations presented in this guideline.

Conclusion

Courage

As the old man walked the beach at dawn, he noticed a young woman ahead of him picking up starfish and flinging them into the sea. Finally catching up with the youth, he asked her why she was doing this. The answer was that the stranded starfish would die if left to the morning sun.

"But the beach goes on for miles and there are millions of starfish," countered the old man. "How can your effort make any difference?"

The young woman looked at the starfish in her hand and threw it to safety in the waves. "It makes a difference to this one," she said.

(Adapted from *The Unexpected Universe*
by Loren Eiseley. Copyright 1969, Harcourt Brace,
New York. Used with permission.)

Too easily can we become overwhelmed by the enormity of the AIDS pandemic. The numbers of patients and their constant needs have caused many to become paralyzed into inactivity and lulled into indifference. Like the old man, many ask "Why bother?"

For the sake of every individual living with HIV, we must focus on what each one of us can do. Each person can make a difference. Believing this, we are empowered to cope with the larger whole.

References

Aboulker JP, Swart AM. Preliminary analysis of the Concorde trial [letter]. Lancet 1993;341(8849):889-90.

AIDS and Adolescents' Network of New York. HIV antibody counseling and testing for adolescents: policy recommendations and practical guidelines. New York: Author; 1992.

Alcabes P, Vossenas P, Cohen R et al. Compliance with isoniazid prophylaxis in jail. Am Rev Respir Dis 1989;140:1194-7.

American Academy of Ophthalmology. Preferred practice pattern: comprehensive adult. San Francisco: Author; 1992 Jun 13.

American College of Obstetricians and Gynecologists. Cervical cytology: evaluation and management of abnormalities, Technical Bulletin No. 81. Washington: Author; 1989.

American College of Obstetricians and Gynecologists. Human immuno-deficiency virus infections, Technical Bulletin No. 165. Washington: Author; 1992 Mar.

Andrews R, Preston B, Howell E, Keyes, M. A comparative analysis of AIDS service demonstration projects in Los Angeles, Miami, New York and San Francisco: a report submitted to the Health Resources and Services Administration. New York: SysteMetrics/McGraw Hill, Inc.; 1989 Oct 16.

Andrulis DP, Weslowski VB, Gage LS. The 1987 US Hospital AIDS survey. JAMA 1989;262:784-94.

Arras JD. AIDS and reproductive decisions: having children in fear and trembling. Milbank Q 1990;68(3):353-82.

Association for Research on Vision and Ophthalmology. The development of cottonwool spots in HIV-positive patients. Invest Ophthalmol Vis Sci [abstract issue] 1990 Apr 29-May 4;31(4):142.

Atkins JN. Maternal plasma concentration of pyridoxal phosphate during pregnancy: adequacy of vitamin B6 supplementation during isoniazid therapy. Am Rev Resp Dis 1982;126:714-6.

Auerbach J (Massachusetts AIDS Director; Vice-Chairman of the National Association of State and Territorial AIDS Directors). Testimony before the Senate Labor and Human Resources Committee. Washington; 1992 Jun 2.

Balacco GC, Angarano G, Moramarco A et al. Ocular manifestations in HIV-seropositive patients. Ann Ophthalmol 1990;22(5):173-6.

Banerjee C, Cromwell G, Furth P. Tuberculin skin testing in HIV infected persons [abstract W.B.274]. Int Conf AIDS; 1989 Jun 4-9. p. 397.

Bash MC, Robb M, Ascher D et al. T-cell subsets and disease status in HIV-infected children [abstract F.B.467]. Int Conf AIDS; 1990 Jun 20-23. p. 194.

Bayer R, Toomey KE. HIV prevention and the two faces of partner notification. Am J Public Health 1992;82:1158-64.

Becherer PR, Smiley ML, Matthews TJ et al. Human immunodeficiency virus-1 disease progression in hemophiliacs. Am J Hematol 1990 Jul;34(3):204-9.

Begg M, Phelan J, Mitchell-Lewis D et al. Relationship of lymphocyte markers to occurrence of oral lesions in HIV infection. J Dent Res 1992;71:561.

Bell TA, Hein K. Adolescents and sexually transmitted diseases. In: Holmes KK, March PA, Sparling PF et al., editors. Sexually transmitted diseases. New York: McGraw Hill; 1984. p. 73-84.

Belman AL. AIDS and pediatric neurology. Neurol Clin 1990;8:571-603.

Belman AL, Ultmann MH, Horoupian D et al. Neurological complications in infants and children with acquired immunodeficiency syndrome. Ann Neurol 1985;18(5):560-6.

Benjamin AE. Long term care and AIDS: perspectives from experience with the elderly. Milbank Q 1988;66:415-43.

Benjamin AR, Lee PR, Solkowitz, SN. Case management of persons with acquired immunodeficiency syndrome in San Francisco. Health Care Financ Rev 1988 Dec;Spec:69-74.

Bennett JC. Inclusion of women in clinical trials-policy population subgroups. N Engl J Med 1993;329(4):288-92.

Bernstein LJ, Bye MR, Rubinstein A. Prognostic factors and life expectancy in children with acquired immunodeficiency syndrome and Pneumocystis carinii pneumonia. Am J Dis Child 1989;143:775-8.

Berry CD, Hooton TM, Collier AC, Lukehart SA. Neurologic relapse after benzathine penicillin therapy for secondary syphilis in a patient with HIV infection. N Engl J Med 1987;316(25):1587-9.

Blanche S, Caniglia M, Fischer A et al. Zidovudine therapy in children with acquired immunodeficiency syndrome. Am J Med 1988 Jul-Sep;85(2A):203-7.

Blanche S, Rouzioux C, Moscato ML et al. A prospective study of infants born to women seropositive for human immunodeficiency virus type 1. HIV infection in newborns. N Engl J Med 1989 Jun;320(25):1643-8.

Blanche S, Tardieu M, Duliege A et al. Longitudinal study of 94 symptomatic infants with perinatally acquired human immunodeficiency virus infection. Am J Dis Child 1990 Nov;114(11):1210-5.

Blatt SP, Donovan D, Freeman T et al. Cutaneous delayed-type hypersensitivity DTH skin testing in HIV-infected patients: implications for diagnosis and chemoprophylaxis of tuberculosis. Int Conf AIDS; 1991 Jun 16-21. 1:464, 2:460.

Blatt SP, Hendrix CW, Butzin A et al. Delayed-type hypersensitivity skin testing predicts progression to AIDS in HIV-infected patients. Ann Int Med 1993 Aug;119(3):177-184.

Blomberg PS, Flynn N. Comprehensive HIV case management protocols for 26 northern California counties [abstract W.B.F.63]. Int Conf AIDS; 1989 Jun 4-9. p. 362.

Boland M, Tasker M, Evans P, Keresztes J. Helping children with AIDS: the role of the child welfare worker. Public Health 1987;23:23-9.

Bolski E, Hunt RJ. The prevalence of AIDS-associated oral lesions in a cohort of patients with hemophilia. Oral Surg Oral Med Oral Pathol 1988;65(4):406-10.

Bonebrake CR, Noller KL, Loehnen CP et al. Routine chest roentgenography in pregnancy. JAMA 1978;240(25):2747-8.

Bradbeer C. Is infection with HIV a risk factor for cervical intraepithelial neoplasia? Lancet 1987;11:1277-8.

Brennan TA. AIDS and the limits of confidentiality: the physician's duty to warn contacts of seropositive individuals. J Gen Intern Med 1989 May-Jun;4(3):242-6.

Briggs GG, Bodendorfer TW, Freeman RK, Yaffe SJ. Drugs in pregnancy and lactation. A reference guide to fetal and neonatal risk. Baltimore: Williams & Wilkins; 1983.

Briggs RM, Paavonen J. Cervical intraepithelial neoplasia. In: Holmes KK, Mardh PA, Sparling PF, Wiesner PJ, editors. Sexually transmitted diseases. New York: McGraw-Hill; 1984. p. 609-11.

Brouwers P, Belman AL, Epstein LG. Central nervous system involvement: manifestations and evaluation. In: Pizzo PA, Wilfert CM, editors. Pediatric AIDS: the challenge of HIV infection in infants, children, and adolescents. Baltimore: Williams & Wilkins; 1991. p. 318-35.

Brouwers P, Moss H, Wolters P et al. Effect of continuous-infusion zidovudine therapy on neuropsychologic functioning in children with symptomatic human immunodeficiency virus infection. J Pediatr 1990;117:980-5.

Brown S, Barton S, Cutland D et al. A study of disclosure of HIV antibody positive status: relationship to use of services and need for support [abstract S.C.652]. Int Conf AIDS; 1990 Jun 20-23. p. 252.

Brudney K, Dobkin J. Resurgent tuberculosis in New York City. Am Rev Respir Dis 1991;144:745-9.

Burke DS, Brundage JF, Goldenbaum M et al. Human immunodeficiency virus infections in teenagers. JAMA 1990;263(15):2074-7.

Burr CK, Emery J. Speaking with children and families about HIV-infections. In: Pizzo PA, Wilfert CM, editors. Pediatric AIDS: the challenge of HIV infection in infants, children and adolescents. 2nd ed. Baltimore: Williams & Wilkins; in press.

Butler KM, Husson RN, Balis FM et al. Dideoxyinosine in children with symptomatic human immunodeficiency virus infection. N Engl J Med 1991;324(3):137-44.

111

Byers J. AIDS in children: effects on neurological development and implications for the future. J Spec Educ 1989;23:1.

Byrne MA, Taylor-Robinson D, Munday PE, Harris JRW. The common occurrence of human papillomavirus infection and intraepithelial neoplasia in women infected by HIV. AIDS 1989;3:379-82.

Canessa PA, Fasano L, Lavecchia MA et al. Tuberculin skin test in asymptomatic HIV seropositive carriers [letter, comment]. Chest 1989;96(5):1215-6.

Capiluto EL, Piette J, White BA, Fleishman J. Perceived need for dental care among persons living with acquired immunodeficiency syndrome. Med Care 1991;29:745-54.

Capitman JA, Haskins B, Bernstein J. Case management approaches in community-oriented long term care demonstrations. Gerontologist 1986 Aug;26(4):398-404.

Caplan R. AIDS and employment in New Jersey: private employers and public policy. In: Gostin LO, editor. AIDS and the health care system. New Haven: Yale University Press; 1990.

Carr A. Trimethoprim-sulfamethoxazole appears more effective than aerosolized pentamidine as secondary prophylaxis against Pneumocystis carinii pneumonia in patients with AIDS. AIDS 1992;6:165-71.

Carr A, Tindell B, Brew BJ et al. Low-dose trimethoprim-sulfamethoxazole prophylaxis for toxoplasmic encephalitis in patients with AIDS. Ann Intern Med 1992;117:106-11.

Casswell DG. Disclosure by a physician of AIDS-related patient information: an ethical and legal dilemma. Can Bar Rev 1989 Jun;68(2):225-58.

Centers for Disease Control. American Thoracic Society. Treatment of tuberculosis and tuberculosis infection in adults and children. Am Rev Resp Dis 1986;134:355-63.

Centers for Disease Control. Classification system for human immunodeficiency virus (HIV) infection in children under 13 years of age. MMWR 1987 Apr;36(15):225-35.

Centers for Disease Control. Recommendations for diagnosing and treating syphilis in HIV-infected patients. MMWR 1988 Oct;37(39):600-8.

Centers for Disease Control. Tuberculosis and human immunodeficiency virus infection: recommendations of the Advisory Committee for the Elimination of Tuberculosis (ACET). MMWR 1989 Apr;38(14):236-50.

Centers for Disease Control. Guidelines for preventing the transmission of tuberculosis in health care settings, with special focus on HIV-related issues. MMWR 1990 Dec;39(RR-17):1-29.

Centers for Disease Control. Guidelines for prophylaxis against Pneumocystis carinii pneumonia for children infected with human immunodeficiency virus. MMWR 1991a Mar;40(RR-2):1-13.

Centers for Disease Control. Purified protein derivative (PPD)-tuberculin anergy and HIV infection: guidelines for anergy testing and management of anergic persons at risk of tuberculosis. MMWR 1991b Apr;40(RR-5):37-43.

Centers for Disease Control. 1993 revised classification system for HIV infection and expanded surveillance case definition for AIDS among adolescents and adults. MMWR 1992a Dec;41(RR-17):1-19.

Centers for Disease Control. Guidelines for the performance of CD4+ T-cell determinations in persons with human immunodeficiency virus infection. MMWR 1992b May;41(RR-8):1-17.

Centers for Disease Control. Guidelines for prophylaxis against Pneumocystis carinii for adults and adolescents infected with human immunodeficiency virus. MMWR 1992c Apr;41(RR-4):1-11.

Centers for Disease Control. Prevention and control of tuberculosis in U.S. communities with at-risk populations: recommendations of the Advisory Council for the elimination of tuberculosis. MMWR 1992d;41(RR-5):1-11.

Centers for Disease Control. National action plan to combat multidrug-resistant tuberculosis; meeting the challenge of multidrug-resistant tuberculosis: summary of a conference; management of persons exposed to multidrug-resistant tuberculosis. MMWR 1992e Jun;41(RR-11):1-71.

Centers for Disease Control. HIV/AIDS surveillance report. MMWR 1992f Apr;1-18.

Centers for Disease Control. HIV instruction and selected HIV risk behaviors among high school students: United States, 1989-1991. MMWR 1992g;41(46):866-8.

Centers for Disease Control. Treatment of tuberculosis: recommendations of the Advisory Council for the elimination of tuberculosis. MMWR 1993.

Chamberlain MC, Nichols SL, Chase CH. Pediatric AIDS: comparative cranial MRI and CT scans. Pediatr Neurol 1991;7(5):357-60.

Christiano A, Susser I. Knowledge and perceptions of HIV infection among homeless pregnant women. J Nurse Midwifery 1989 Nov-Dec;34(6):318-22.

Chu SY, Buehler MJ, Oxtoby MJ, Kilborne BW. Impact of the HIV epidemic on mortality in children, United States. Pediatrics 1991;87:806-10.

Coates TJ, Lo B. Counseling patients seropositive for human immunodeficiency virus. An approach for medical practice. West J Med 1990 Dec;153(6):629-34.

Cohen J, Nardell E. Anergy in intravenous drug users (IVDUs); prevalence, influence of HIV status, sex [abstract F.B.502]. Int Conf AIDS; 1990 Jun 20-23. p. 203.

Collins FM. Antituberculous immunity: new solutions to an old problem. Rev Infect Dis 1991;13(5):940-50.

Combs DL, O'Brien RJ, Geiter LJ. USPHS tuberculosis short-course chemotherapy trial 21: effectiveness, toxicity, and acceptability. Ann Intern Med 1990;112(6):397-406.

Congressional Research Service. Medicaid source book: background data and analysis. Washington: 100th Congress, 2d session; 1988 Nov.

Connor E, Bagarazzi M, McSherry G et al. Clinical and laboratory correlates of Pneumocystis carinii pneumonia in children infected with HIV. JAMA 1991 Apr;265(13):1693-7.

Conte JE, Chernoff D, Feigal DW et al. Intravenous or inhaled pentamidine for treating Pneumocystis carinii pneumonia in AIDS. Ann Intern Med 1990;113:203-9.

Conti M, Muggiasca ML, Conti E. Human immunodeficiency virus infection and cervical intraepithelial neoplasia. Cervix 1989;7:215-29.

Cooley TP, Kunches LM, Saunders CA et al. Treatment of AIDS in AIDS-related complex with 2', 3' dideoxyinosine given once daily. Rev Infect Dis 1990 Jul-Aug;12(Suppl 5):5552-60.

Cooney TG. Clinical management of the complications of HIV infection. J Gen Intern Med 1991;6(Suppl 1):S12-8.

Cooper DA, Gatell JM, Kroon S et al. Zidovudine in persons with asymptomatic HIV infection and CD4+ cell counts greater than 400 per cubic millimeter. N Engl J Med 1993;329(5):297-303.

Cotton P. Is there still too much extrapolation from data on middle-aged white men? JAMA 1990;263:1049-50.

Crocker AC. Developmental services for children with HIV infection. Ment Retard 1989;27:223-5.

Dalakas MC, Pezeshkpour GH. Neuromuscular diseases associated with human immunodeficiency virus infection. Ann Neurol 1988;23(Suppl):S38-48.

Daley CL, Small PM, Schecter GF et al. An outbreak of tuberculosis with accelerated progression among persons infected with human immunodeficiency virus: an analysis using restriction-fragment-length polymorphisms. N Engl J Med 1992;326(4):231-5.

Davis MJ. Oral health care in pediatrics AIDS. NY State Dent J 1990;56:25-7.

DeCarli C, Fugate L, Falloon J et al. Brain growth and cognitive improvement in children with human immunodeficiency virus-induced encephalopathy after 6 months of continuous infusion zidovudine therapy. J Acquir Immune Defic Syndr 1991 Jan-Jun;4(1):585-92.

Dehovitz JA. The increasing role of primary care in the management of HIV-infected patients. NY State J Med 1990;119-21.

deMartino M, Tovo P-A, Galli L et al. Prognostic significance of immunological change in 675 infants perinatally exposed to human immunodeficiency virus. J Pediatr 1991;119(5):702-9.

Denny T, Yogev R, Gelman R et al. Lymphocyte subsets in healthy children during the first four years of life. JAMA 1992;267(11):1484-8.

DeRossi A, Ades AE, Mammano F et al. Antigen detection, virus culture, polymerase chain reaction and in vitro antibody production in the diagnosis of vertically transmitted HIV-1 infection. AIDS 1991;5(1):15-20.

Dickson DW, Belman AL, Kim TS. Spinal cord pathology in pediatric acquired immunodeficiency syndrome. Neurology 1989;39:227-35.

Dodd CL, Greenspan D, Katz MH et al. Oral candidiasis in HIV infection: pseudomembranous and erythematous candidiasis show similar rates of progression to AIDS. AIDS 1992;5:1339-43.

Dodd CL, Greenspan D, Westenhouse JL, Katz MH. Xerostomia associated with 2', 3' dideoxyinosine (ddI) therapy [letter]. Lancet 1992;740:790.

Dowell ME, Ross PG, Musher DM et al. Response of latent syphilis or neurosyphilis to ceftriaxone therapy in persons infected with human immunodeficiency virus. Am J Med 1992;93:481-8.

Drew WL. Cytomegalovirus virus infection in patients with AIDS. Clin Infect Dis 1992;14:608-15.

Durst M, Gissmann L, Ikenberg H, zur Hausen H. A papillomavirus DNA from a cervical carcinoma and its prevalence in cancer biopsy samples from different geographic regions. Proc Natl Acad Sci USA 1983 Jun;80(12):3812-5.

Edlin R, Tokars JI, Grieco MH, Crawford JJT. An outbreak of multidrug resistant tuberculosis among hospitalized patients with the acquired immunodeficiency syndrome. N Engl J Med 1992;326:1514-21.

Edwards JR, Ulrich PP, Weintrub PS et al. Polymerase chain reaction compared with concurrent viral cultures for rapid identification of human immunodeficiency virus infection among high risk infants and children. J Pediatr 1989;115(2):200-3.

Eisenach KD, Sifford MD, Cave MD et al. Detection of mycobacterium tuberculosis in sputum samples using a polymerase chain reaction. Am Rev Resp Dis 1991;144:1160-3.

El-Sadr W, Capps L. The challenge of minority recruitment in clinical trials for AIDS. JAMA 1992;267(7):954-7.

Elmslie T, Shearman J, Busing N. HIV antibody testing by Canadian general practitioners and family physicians [abstract Th.E.P.10]. Int Conf AIDS; 1989 Jun 4-9. p. 874.

Emlet, CA. Coordinating county-based services for the frail elderly: a tri-departmental approach. J Gerontol Soc Work 1982 8(1):5-13.

Employee Benefit Research Institute. Sources of health insurance and characteristics of the uninsured: analysis of the March 1991 current population survey; EBRI Issue Brief No. 123. Washington: Author; 1992.

English A. In: DiClemente R, editor. AIDS in adolescents. Newbury Park, CA: Sage Publications; 1992.

Epstein LG, DiCarlo FJ, Joshi VV et al. Primary lymphoma of the central nervous system in children with acquired immunodeficiency syndrome. Pediatrics 1988;82(3):355-63.

Epstein LG, Goudsmit J, Paul DA et al. Expression of human immunodeficiency virus in cerebrospinal fluid of children with progressive encephalopathy. Ann Neurol 1989;21(4):397-401.

Epstein LG, Sharer LR, Oleske JM et al. Neurologic manifestations of HIV infection in children. Pediatrics 1986;78(4):678-87.

European Collaborative Study. Mother-to-child transmission of HIV infection. Lancet 1988;2:639-42.

European Collaborative Study. Neurologic signs in young children with human immunodeficiency virus infection. Pediatr Infect Dis J 1990;9(6):402-6.

European Collaborative Study. Children born to women with HIV-1 infection: natural history and risks of transmission. Lancet 1991;337(8736):253-60.

Fahey JL, Taylor JM, Detels R et al. The prognostic value of cellular and serologic markers in infection with human immunodeficiency virus type 1 [see comments]. N Engl J Med 1990 Jan;322(3):166-72.

Fauci AS. The human immunodeficiency virus: infectivity and mechanisms of pathogenesis. Science 1988;239:617-22.

Fauci AS. AIDS: challenges to basic and clinical biomedical research. Acad Med 1989;64:115-9.

Feigal DW, Katz MH, Greenspan D et al. The prevalence of oral lesions in HIV-infected homosexual and bisexual men: three San Francisco epidemiology cohorts. AIDS 1991;5:519-25.

Feingold AR, Vermund SH, Burk RD et al. Cervical cytologic abnormalities and papillomavirus in women infected with human immunodeficiency virus. J Acquir Immune Defic Syndr 1990;3:896-903.

Feldblum PJ, Fortney JA. Condoms, spermicides and the transmission of human immunodeficiency virus: a review of the literature. Am J Public Health 1988;78(1):52-4.

Feldsman JL, Tucker MS, Leifer JC et al. Legal issues in pediatric HIV practice: a handbook for health care providers. Newark NJ: National Pediatric HIV Resource Center; 1992.

Ficarra G, Person AM, Silverman S. Kaposi's sarcoma of the oral cavity: a study of 134 patients with a review of the pathogenesis, epidemiology, clinical aspects and treatment. Oral Surg Oral Med Oral Pathol 1988;66:543-50.

Fischl MA, Dickinson GM, La Voie L. Safety and efficacy of sulfamethoxazole and trimethoprim chemoprophylaxis for Pneumocystis carinii pneumonia in AIDS. JAMA 1988 Feb;259(8):1185-9.

Fischl M, Galpin JE, Levine JD et al. Recombinant human erythropoietin for patients with AIDS treated with zidovudine. N Engl J Med 1990;322:1488-93.

Fischl MA, Richman DD, Grieco MH. The efficacy of azidothymidine (AZT) in the treatment of patients with AIDS and AIDS related complex. A double-blind placebo-controlled trial. N Engl J Med 1987;317:185-91.

References

Fischl MA, Uttamchandani RB, Daikos GL et al. An outbreak of tuberculosis caused by multiple-drug-resistant tubercle bacilli among patients with HIV infection. Ann Intern Med 1992 Aug;117(3)177-81.

Fisher E, Nussbaum J, Frasier K. Results of screening for cytomegalovirus (CMV) retinitis [abstract 2155]. Int Conf AIDS; 1990 Jun 20-23. p. 392.

Flaskerud JH, Rush CE. AIDS and traditional health beliefs and practices of black women. Nurs Res 1989 Jul-Aug;38(4):210-5.

Food and Drug Administration. General considerations for the clinical evaluation of drugs. Washington: Government Printing Office (US); 1977.

Food and Drug Administration. FDA guideline on women in clinical trials. Rockville (MD): Public Health Service; 1993 Jul 21.

Forrest J. American women's sexual behavior and exposure to risk of sexually transmitted diseases. Fam Plann Perspect 1992;24(6):244-54.

Fortin C, Boyer R, Duval B et al. Physician's attitudes towards HIV screening and contact tracing in the province of Quebec [abstract 3052]. Int Conf AIDS; 1990 Jun 20-23. p. 415.

Frederick T, Mascola L, Evans M et al. Clinical and immunological features associated with pediatric HIV infection in Los Angeles county, California, USA [abstract T.B.P.161]. Int Conf AIDS; 1989 Jun 4-9. p. 313.

Freedberg KA, Tosteson AN, Cohen CJ, Cotton DJ. Primary prophylaxis for Pneumocystis carinii pneumonia in HIV-infected people with CD4 counts below 200/mm^3: a cost-effectiveness analysis. J Acquir Immune Defic Syndr 1991;4(5):521-31.

Freeman WR, Chen A, Henderly DE et al. Prevalence and significance of acquired immunodeficiency syndrome-related retinal microvasculopathy. Am J Ophthalmol 1989;107(3):229-35.

Futterman D, Hein K. Medical management of adolescents. In: Pizzo PA, Wilfert CM, editors. Pediatric AIDS. Baltimore: Williams & Wilkins; 1990. p. 546-60.

Futterman D, Hein K. Medical care of HIV-infected adolescents. AIDS Clin Care 1992;4:95-8.

Girard PM, Landman R, Gaudebout C et al. Dapsone-pyrimethamine compared with aerosolized pentamidine as primary prophylaxis against Pneumocystis carinii pneumonia and toxoplasmosis in HIV infection. N Engl J Med 1993 May 27;328(21):1514-20.

Goedert JJ, Duliege AM, Amos CI et al. High risk of HIV-1 infection for first-born twins. The International Registry of HIV-Exposed Twins. Lancet 1991 Dec;338(8781):1471-5.

Goldschmidt RH, Legg JJ. Counseling patients about HIV test results. J Am Board Fam Pract 1991 Sep-Oct;4:361-3.

Good JT, Iseman MD, Davidson PT et al. Tuberculosis in association with pregnancy. Am J Obstet Gynecol 1981;140:492-8.

117

Goodman PC. Pulmonary tuberculosis in patients with acquired immunodeficiency syndrome. J Thorac Imaging 1990;5(2):38-45.

Gourevitch MN, Selwyn PA, Davenny K et al. Effects of HIV infection on the serologic manifestations and response to treatment of syphilis in intravenous drug users. Ann Intern Med 1993;118:350-5.

Graham NMH, Nelson KE, Solomon L et al. Prevalence of tuberculin positivity and skin test anergy in HIV-1-seropositive and seronegative intravenous drug users. JAMA 1992;267:369-73.

Graham NM, Zeger SL, Park LP et al. The effects on survival of early treatment of human immunodeficiency virus infection. N Engl J Med 1992 Apr;326(16):1037-42.

Grange JM. The rapid diagnosis of paucibacillary tuberculosis. Tubercle 1989;70(1)1-4.

Greenspan D, de Villiers EM, Greenspan JS et al. Unusual HPV types in oral warts in association with HIV infection. J Oral Pathol 1988 Nov;17:482-8.

Greenspan D, Greenspan JS. Management of the oral lesions of HIV infection. J Am Dent Assoc 1991;26-32.

Greenspan D, Greenspan JS, Conant M et al. Oral "hairy" leucoplakia in male homosexuals: evidence of association with both papillomavirus and a herpes-group virus. Lancet 1984 Oct;2(8407):831-4.

Greenspan D, Greenspan JS, Overby G et al. Risk factors for rapid progression from hairy leukoplakia to AIDS: a nested case-control study. J Acquir Immune Defic Syndr 1991;4(7):652-8.

Greenspan JS, Barr CE, Sciubba JJ et al. Oral manifestations of HIV infection: definitions, diagnostic criteria and principles of therapy. Oral Surg Oral Med Oral Pathol 1992;73:142-4.

Greenspan JS, Greenspan D, Lennett ET et al. Replication of Epstein-Barr virus within the epithelial cells of oral "hairy" leukoplakia, an AIDS associated lesion. N Engl J Med 1985;313(25):1564-71.

Gregory N, Sanchez M., Buchness MR. The spectrum of syphilis in patients with human immunodeficiency virus infection. J Am Acad Dermatol 1990;22(6):1061-7.

Groopman JE, Mitsuyasu RT, DeLeo MJ et al. Effect of recombinant human granulocyte-macrophage colony-stimulating factor on myelopoiesis in the acquired immunodeficiency syndrome. N Engl J Med 1989;317(10):593-658.

Gupta A, Ravipati M, Slade H. Disease progression and effect of zidovudine (AZT) in pediatric AIDS [abstract T.B.P.354]. Int Conf AIDS; 1989 Jun 4-9. p. 329.

Gupta P, Brady M, Raabe M, Urbach A. Detection of human immunodeficiency virus by virus culture and polymerase chain reaction in children born to seropositive mothers. J Acquir Immune Defic Syndr 1991;4:1004-6.

Haas JS, Bolan G, Larsen SA et al. Sensitivity of treponemal tests for detecting prior treated syphilis during human immunodeficiency virus infection. J Infect Dis 1990;162(4):862-6.

Haiken H, Hernandez M, Mintz M, Boland M. School aged HIV-infected children and access to education [abstract Th.D.849]. Int Conf AIDS 1990 Jun;6(1):338.

Halpert R, Fruchter RG, Sedlis A et al. Human papillomavirus and lower genital neoplasia in renal transplant patients. Obstet Gynecol 1986;68(2):251-8.

Hamilton JD, Hartigan PH, Simberkoff MD et al. A controlled trial of early versus late treatment with zidovudine in symptomatic human immunodeficiency virus infection. Results of the Veterans Affairs Cooperative Study. N Engl J Med 1992;326(7):437-43.

Haney PJ, Yale-Loehr AJ, Nussbaum AR, Gellad FE. Imaging of infants and children with AIDS [rev. article]. Am J Roentgenol 1989;152:1033-41.

Hanson CA, Reichman LB. Tuberculosis skin testing and preventive therapy. Semin Respir Infect 1989;4(3):182-8.

Harder and Kibbe Research. Review of case management and HIV; 1991 Dec. Unpublished manuscript.

Hardy WD, Feinberg J, Finkelstein DM et al. A controlled trial of trimethoprim-sulfamethoxazole or aerosolized pentamidine for secondary prophylaxis of Pneumocystis carinii pneumonia in patients with the acquired immunodeficiency syndrome. N Engl J Med 1992;327:1842-8.

Harmon R (Administrator, Health Resources and Services Administration). Testimony before the Senate Labor and Human Resources Committee concerning the implementation of the Ryan White CARE Act. 1992 Jun.

Harris M, Bergman H. Case management with the chronically mentally ill: a clinical perspective. Am J Orthopsychiatry 1987;57:296-302.

Haverkos HW. Assessment of therapy for Pneumocystis carinii pneumonia: PCP therapy project group. Am J Med 1984;76:501-8.

Hazard M, Shervington W, Stroud F et al. Meeting the health care needs of minorities with HIV infection [abstract D.661]. Int Conf AIDS; 1989 Jun 4-9. p. 801.

Hein K. Mandatory HIV testing of youth: a lose-lose proposition. JAMA 1991;266(2):2430-1.

Hein K, Futterman D. Guideline for the care of children and adolescents with HIV infection: Medical management in HIV-infected adolescents. J Pediatr 1991 Jul;119(1 Pt 2):518-520.

Hellinger, F. Forecasts of the costs of medical care for persons with HIV: 1992-1995. Inquiry 1992 Fall;29:356-65.

Henderly DE, Jampol LM. Diagnosis and treatment of cytomegalovirus retinitis. J Acquir Immune Defic Syndr 1991;4(Suppl 1):S6-10.

Henry MJ, Stanley MW, Cruikshank S, Carson L. Association of human immunodeficiency virus-induced immunosuppression with human papillomavirus infection and cervical intraepithelial neoplasia. Am J Obstet Gynecol 1989;160:352-3.

Heyes MP, Robinow D, Lane C, Markey SP. Cerebrospinal fluid quinolinic acid concentrations are increased in acquired immunodeficiency syndrome. Ann Neurol 1989;26(2):275-7.

Hicks CB, Benson PM, Lupton GP, Tramont EC. Seronegative secondary syphilis, the human immunodeficiency virus (HIV), and Kaposi's sarcoma. Ann Intern Med 1987;107(6):946.

Hingson RW, Strunin L, Berlin BM, Heeren T. Beliefs about AIDS, use of alcohol and drugs, and unprotected sex among Massachusetts adolescents. Am J Public Health 1990;80(3)195-299.

Hirschel B, Lazzarin A, Chopard P et al. A controlled study of inhaled pentamidine for primary prevention of Pneumocystis carinii pneumonia. N Engl J Med 1991 Apr;324(16):1079-83.

Holman S, Berthaud M, Sunderland A et al. Women infected with human immunodeficiency virus: counseling and testing during pregnancy. Semin Perinatol 1989;13(1)7-15.

Holtom PD, Larsen RA, Leal ME, Leedom JM. Prevalence of neurosyphilis in human immunodeficiency virus-infected patients with latent syphilis. Am J Med 1992 Jul;93(1):9-12.

Holtzman D, Anderson JE, Kann L et al. HIV instruction, HIV knowledge, and drug injection among high school students in the United States. Am J Public Health 1991;81:1596-1601.

Holtzman D, Mathis MP, Kann L et al. Trends in HIV-related instructions and behaviors among high school students in the United States; 1989-1991 [abstract P.O.D. 5114]. Int AIDS Conf; 1992. p. 406.

Honnard R. The chronically mentally ill in the community. In: Weil, M, Karls, JM, editors. Case management in human services practice. San Francisco: Josey-Bass; 1985. p. 204-232.

Hook EW III. Syphilis and HIV infection. J Infect Dis 1989;160(3):530-4.

Hook EW III, Marra CM. Acquired syphilis in adults. N Engl J Med 1992;326(16):1060-9.

House Select Committee. A decade of denial: teens and AIDS in America. A report of the Select Committee on Children, Youth and Families; House of Representatives, 1992 May; 102d Congress, 2d Session.

Hu DJ, Heyward WL, Byers RH et al. HIV infection and breast feeding: policy implications through a decision analysis model. AIDS 1992;68:1505-13.

Hughes WT, Kuhn S, Chaudhary S et al. Successful chemoprophylaxis for Pneumocystis carinii pneumonitis. N Engl J Med 1977 Dec;297(26):1419-26.

Hunter ND. Complications of gender: women and HIV disease. In: Hunter ND, Rubenstein WB, editors. AIDS agenda: emerging issues in civil rights. New York: The New Press; 1992.

Hutchinson CM, Rompalo AM, Reichart CA, Hook EW III. Characteristics of patients with syphilis attending Baltimore STD clinics: multiple high risk subgroups and interactions with human immunodeficiency virus infection. Arch Intern Med 1991 Mar;151(3):511-6.

Hutchinson M, Kurth A. "I need to know that I have a choice..." A study of women, HIV and reproductive decision-making. AIDS Patient Care 1991 Feb;5:17-25.

Hutto C, Parks WP, Lai S et al. A hospital-based prospective study of perinatal infection with human immunodeficiency virus type 1. J Pediatr 1991 Mar;118(3):347-53.

Indyk D, Wade K. Integrating community based and hospital based case management. Focus: A Guide to AIDS Research and Counseling 1992 Sep;7(10):1-4.

Insler MS. AIDS and the other sexually transmitted diseases and the eye. Orlando (FL): Grune and Stratton, Inc.; 1987.

Institute of Medicine. Clinical practice guidelines: directions for a new program. Field MJ, Lohr CL, editors. Washington: National Academy Press; 1990.

Intergovernmental Health Policy Project. State financing for AIDS: options and trends. Intergovernmental AIDS Rep 1990 Mar-Apr;3(1):1-12.

Intergovernmental Health Policy Project. National survey of state-only HIV funds. Intergovernmental AIDS Rep 1991 Nov;4:1-16.

Italian Multicentre Study. Epidemiology, clinical features, and prognostic factors of pediatric HIV infection. Lancet 1988 Nov;2(8619):1043-6.

Jabs DA, Green WR, Fox R et al. Ocular manifestations of acquired immune deficiency syndrome. Ophthalmology 1989;96(7):1092-9.

Jaffe HW. Management of reactive serology. In Sexually transmitted diseases. Holmes KK, March PA, Sparling PF et al., editors. New York; McGraw-Hill; 1984. p. 313-7.

James ME, Rubin CP, Willis SE. Drug abuse and psychiatric findings in HIV-seropositive pregnant patients. Gen Hosp Psychiatry 1991 Jan;13(1):4-8.

Jellinek PS. Case-managing AIDS. Issues Sci Technol 1988 Summer;4(4):142-3.

Jemmott JB, Jemmott LS, Fong GT. Reductions in HIV risk-associated sexual behaviors among black male adolescents: effects of an AIDS prevention intervention. Am J Public Health 1992;82(3):372-7.

Jendis JB, Tomasik Z, Hunziker U et al. Evaluation of diagnostic tests for HIV infection in infants born to HIV-infected mothers in Switzerland. AIDS 1988;2(4):273-9.

Johns DR, Tierney M, Felsenstein D. Alteration in the natural history of neurosyphilis by concurrent infection with the human immunodeficiency virus. N Engl J Med 1987;316(25):1569-72.

Johnson JC, Burnett AF, Willet GD et al. High frequency of latent and clinical human papillomavirus cervical infections in immunocompromised human immunodeficiency virus-infected women. Obstet Gynecol 1992;79(3):321-7.

Johnson MP, Coberly JS, Clermont HE, Chaisson RE. Tuberculin skin test reactivity among adults infected with human immunodeficiency virus. J Infect Dis 1992;166:194-8.

Johnson J, Nair P, Hines SE et al. A natural history and serological diagnosis of infants born to human immunodeficiency virus-infected women. Am J Dis Child 1989;143:1147-53.

Jones JL, Wykoff RF, Hollis SL et al. Partner acceptance of health department notification of HIV exposure, South Carolina. JAMA 1990 Sep;264(10):1284-6.

Jordan TJ, Lewit EM, Montgomery RL, Reichman LB. Isoniazid as preventive therapy in HIV-infected intravenous drug abusers. JAMA 1991;265:2987-91.

Kahn G. Dapsone is safe during pregnancy [letter]. J Am Acad Dermatol 1985 Nov;13(5):838-9.

Kahn JO, Lagakos SW, Richman DD et al. A controlled trial comparing continued zidovudine with didanosine in human immunodeficiency virus infection. N Engl J Med 1992;327:581-7.

Kales CP, Mullen JR, Torres RA, Crocco JA. Early predictors of in-hospital mortality for Pneumocystis carinii pneumonia in acquired immunodeficiency syndrome. Arch Intern Med 1987;147:1413-7.

Kane RA. Case management in health care settings. In: Weil M, Karls JM, editors. Case management in human service practice. San Francisco: Josey-Bass; 1985. p. 170-203.

Karan LD. AIDS prevention and chemical dependence treatment needs of women and their children. J Psychoactive Drugs 1989;21(4):395-9.

Kaslow RA. The multicenter AIDS cohort study: rationale, organization, and selected characteristics of the participants. Am J Epidemiol 1987;126:310-8.

Katz DA, Berger JR. Neurosyphilis in acquired immunodeficiency syndrome. Arch Neurol 1989;46:895-8.

Katz MH, Greenspan D, Westenhouse J et al. Progression to AIDS in HIV-infected homosexual and bisexual men with oral candidiasis and hairy leukoplakia: results from three San Francisco epidemiological cohorts. AIDS 1992;6:95-100.

Katz MH, Mastrucci MT, Leggott PJ et al. Prognostic significance of oral lesions in children with perinatally acquired HIV infection. Am J Dis Child; in press.

Kemper P. The evaluation of the national long term care demonstrations. Health Serv Res 1988 Apr;23(1):16-7.

Ketchem I, Berkowitz RJ, McIlveen L et al. Oral findings in HIV-seropositive children. Pediatr Dent 1990 May-Jun;12(3):143-6.

Khouri YF, Mastrucci MT, Hutto C et al. Mycobacterium tuberculosis in children with human immunodeficiency virus type 1 infection. Pediatr Infect Dis J 1992 Nov;11(11):950-5.

Kipke M, Futterman D, Hein K. HIV infection and AIDS during adolescence. Med Clin North Am 1990 Sep;74(5):1149-67.

Klein RS, Quart AM, Small CB. Periodontal disease in heterosexuals with acquired immunodeficiency syndrome. J Periodontol 1991;62:535-40.

Kline AH, Blatter RJ, Lunin M. Transplacental effect of tetracycline on teeth. JAMA 1964;188:178-80.

Knutsen AP, Bouhasin JD, Gioia K, Mueller KB. Zidovudine treatment in adolescent hemophiliac children with HIV infection [abstract T.B.P.253]. Int Conf AIDS; 1989 Jun 4-9. p. 329.

Koonin LM, Ellerbrock TV, Atrash HK et al. Pregnancy-associated deaths due to AIDS in the United States. JAMA 1989 Mar;261(9):1306-9.

Koutsky LA, Holmes KK, Critchlow CW et al. A cohort study of the risk of cervical intraepithelial neoplasia grade 2 or 3 in relation to papillomavirus infection. N Engl J Med 1992;327:1272-8.

Kovacs A, Frederick T, Church J et al. CD4 T-lymphocyte counts and Pneumocystis carinii pneumonia in pediatric HIV infection. JAMA 1991 Apr;265(13):1698-1703.

Krasinski K. Retroviral therapy and clinical trials for HIV-infected children. J Pediatr 1991;119(Suppl 1):S63-8.

Krivine A, Yakudima A, LeMay M et al. A comparative study of virus isolation, polymerase chain reaction and antigen detection in children of mothers infected with immunodeficiency virus. J Pediatr 1990;116(3):372-6.

Ku LC, Sonenstein F, Pleck JH. The association of AIDS education and sex education with sexual behavior and condom use among teenage men. Fam Plann Perspect 1992 May/Jun;24(3):100-7.

Kunins H, Hein K, Futterman D. Guide to adolescent HIV/AIDS program development. J Adolesc Health 1993 July;14(5):22S-24S.

Laga M, Icenogle JP, Marsella R et al. Genital papillomavirus infection and cervical dysplasia-opportunistic complications of HIV infection. Int J Cancer 1992;50(1):45-8.

Lagakos S, Fischl MA, Stein DS et al. Effects of zidovudine therapy in minority and other subpopulations with early HIV infection. JAMA 1991;266(19):2709-12.

Landesman S, Weiblen B, Mendez H et al. Clinical utility of HIV-IgA immunoblot assay in early diagnosis of perinatal HIV infection. JAMA 1991 Dec;266(24):3443-6.

Laure F, Rouzioux C, Veber F et al. Detection of HIV-1 DNA in infants and children by means of the polymerase chain reaction. Lancet 1988 Jul-Sep;3(2):538-42.

Laverda AM, Cogo P, Condini A et al. How frequent and how early does the neurological involvement in HIV-positive children occur? Preliminary results of a prospective study. Childs Nerv Syst 1990;6:406-8.

Lee FK, Nahmias AJ, Lowery S et al. Elispot: a new approach to studying the dynamics of virus-immunosystem intersection for diagnosis and monitoring of HIV infection. AIDS Res Hum Retroviruses 1989;5(5):517-23.

Leggott PJ, Robertson PB, Greenspan D et al. Oral manifestations of primary and acquired immunodeficiency diseases in children. Pediatr Dent 1989;9(2):98-104.

Leibovitz E, Rigaud M, Pollack A et al. Pneumocystis carinii pneumonia in infants with the human immunodeficiency virus with more than 450 CD4 T-lymphocytes per cubic millimeter. N Engl J Med 1990;323(8):531-3.

Leoung GS, Feigal DW, Montgomery AB et al. Aerosolized pentamidine for prophylaxis against Pneumocystis carinii pneumonia. N Engl J Med 1990;323:769-75.

Levine C. Women and HIV/AIDS research: the barriers to equity. Institutional Rev Board 1991;13:18-22.

Levine C, Dubler NN, Levine RJ. Building a new consensus: ethical principles and policies for clinical research on HIV/AIDS. Institutional Rev Board 1991;13:1-17.

Levine RJ. Ethics and regulations of clinical research. 2nd ed. Baltimore: Urban & Schwartzberg; 1986. p. 67-93.

Lipson M. What do you say to a child with AIDS? Hastings Center Report 1993; Mar-Apr; 6-12.

Lo B, Steinbrook RL, Cooke M et al. Voluntary screening for human immunodeficiency virus (HIV) infection: weighing the benefits and harms. Ann Intern Med 1989 May;110(9):727-33.

Long R, Maycher B, Scalcini M, Manfreda J. The chest roentgenogram in pulmonary tuberculosis patients seropositive for human immunodeficiency virus type 1. Chest 1991;99(1):123-7.

Long R, Scalini M, Manfreda J et al. The impact of HIV on the usefulness of sputum smears for the diagnosis of tuberculosis. Am J Public Health 1991;81:1326-8.

Lowe CR. Congenital defects among children born to women under supervision or treatment for pulmonary tuberculosis. Br J Prev Soc Med 1964:18:14.

Lukehart SA, Hook EW III, Baker-Zander SA et al. Invasion of the central nervous system by Treponema pallidum: implications for diagnosis and treatment. Ann Intern Med 1988 Dec;109(11):855-61.

MacDonell KB, Chmiel JS, Poggensee L et al. Predicting progression to AIDS: combined usefulness of CD4 lymphocyte counts and p24 antigenemia [see comments]. Am J Med 1990;89(6):706-12.

Magallon DT. Counseling patients with HIV (human immunodeficiency virus) infections. Med Aspects Hum Sex 1987 Jun;129-47.

Maiman M, Fruchter RG, Serur E, Boyce JG. Prevalence of HIV in a colposcopy clinic. JAMA 1988;260(15):2214-5.

Maiman M, Fruchter RG, Serur E et al. Human immunodeficiency virus infection and cervical neoplasia. Gynecol Oncol 1990;38(3):377-82.

Maiman M, Tarricone N, Vieira J et al. Colposcopic evaluation of human immunodeficiency virus seropositive women. Obstet Gynecol 1991;78(1):84-8.

Mann J, Tarantola DJM, Netter TW, editors. A global report: AIDS in the World. Cambridge (MA): Harvard University Press; 1992. p. 11-108.

Marte C, Cohen M, Fruchter R, Kelly P. PAP test and STD findings in HIV+ women at ambulatory care sites. Am J Obstet Gynecol 1992;166(4):1232-7.

Martin JP. Planning for the future: support for the HIV person. Contin Care 1990 Sep;17-21.

Martin MA, Cox PH, Beck K et al. A comparison of the effectiveness of three regimens in the prevention of Pneumocystis carinii pneumonia in human immunodeficiency virus infected patients. Arch Intern Med 1992;152:523-8.

Martin NL, Long JA, Legg H. Detection of infection with human immunodeficiency virus (HIV) type 1 in infants by an anti-HIV immunoglobulin assay using recombinant proteins. J Pediatr 1991;118:354-8.

Masouredis CM, Katz MH, Greenspan D et al. Prevalence of HIV-associated periodontitis and gingivitis in HIV-infected patients attending an AIDS clinic. J Acquir Immun Defic Syndr 1992;5:479-83.

Mattar S, Broquetas JM, Gea J et al. Serodiagnosis of tuberculosis in patients with antibodies against human immunodeficiency virus. World Conference on Lung Health 1990 May 20-24; Boston. Am Rev Respir Dis 1990;141 (4 part 2):A265.

Mayers DL, McCutchan FE, Sanders-Buell EE et al. Characterization of HIV isolates arising after prolonged zidovudine therapy. J Acquir Immune Defic Syndr 1992;5(8):749-59.

McKinney RE. Antiviral therapy for human immunodeficiency virus infection in children. Pediatr Clin North Am 1991;38(1):133-51.

McKinney RE, Maha MA, Connor EM et al. A multicenter trial of oral zidovudine in children with acquired human immunodeficiency virus disease. N Engl J Med 1991;324(15):1018-25.

McKinney RE, Pizzo PA, Scott GB et al. Safety and tolerance of intermittent intravenous and oral zidovudine therapy in human immunodeficiency virus-infected pediatric patients. J Pediatr 1990;116(4):640-7.

McLeish WM, Palido JS, Holland S et al. The ocular manifestations of syphilis in the human immunodeficiency virus type-1 infected host. Ophthalmology 1990;97(2):196-203.

McSherry G, Berman C, Aguila H et al. Tuberculosis in HIV-infected children in Newark 1981-1992 [abstract 905]. Interscience Conference of Antimicrobial Agents and Chemotherapy; Anaheim (CA); 1992 Oct. p. 261.

Melnick SL, Engel D, Truelove E. Oral mucosal lesions: association with the presence of antibodies to the human immunodeficiency virus. Oral Surg Oral Med Oral Pathol 1989;68:37-43.

Melroe NH. "Duty to warn" vs. "patient confidentiality": the ethical dilemmas in caring for HIV-infected clients. Nurse Pract 1990 Feb;15(2):58, 60, 65.

Meng TC, Fischl MA, Boota AM et al. Combination therapy with zidovudine and dideoxycytidine in patients with advanced human immunodeficiency virus infection. A phase I/II study [see comments]. Ann Intern Med 1992;116(1):13-20.

Merigan TC, Amato DA, Balsley J. Placebo-controlled trial to evaluate zidovudine in treatment of human immunodeficiency virus infection in asymptomatic patients with hemophilia. Blood 1991;78:900-6.

Merkatz RB, Temple R, Sobel S et al. Women in clinical trials of new drugs: a change in Food and Drug Administration policy. N Engl J Med 1993;329(4):292-6.

Merzel C, Crystal S, Sambamoorthi U et al. New Jersey's Medicaid waiver for acquired immune deficiency syndrome. Health Care Finan Rev 1992 Spring;13(3):27-44.

Metroka CE, Braun N, Josefberg H, Jacobs D. Successful chemoprophylaxis for P. carinii pneumonia with dapsone in patients with AIDS and ARC [abstract T.B.O.4]. Int Conf AIDS; 1989 Jun 12-16. p.196.

Michaels D, Levine C. Estimates of the number of motherless youth orphaned by AIDS in the United States. JAMA 1992;268(24):3456-61.

Michaels J, Price RW, Rosenblum MK. Microglia in the giant cell encephalitis of AIDS: proliferation, infection and fusion. Acta Neuropathol 1988;76:373-9.

Miles SA, Balden E, Magpantay L et al. Rapid serologic testing with immune-complex-dissociated HIV p24 antigen for early detection of HIV infection in neonates. N Engl J Med 1993 Feb;328(5):297-302.

Minkoff H. PCP prophylaxis in pregnancy. Am J Obstet Gynecol 1990;162:20-35.

Minkoff HL, DeHovitz JA. Care of women infected with the human immunodeficiency virus. JAMA 1991;266:2253-8.

Minkoff HL, Henderson C, Mendez H et al. Pregnancy outcomes among mothers infected with human immunodeficiency virus and uninfected control subjects. Am J Obstet Gynecol 1990 Nov;163(5 part 1):1598-604.

Minkoff HL, Moreno JD. Drug prophylaxis for human immunodeficiency virus-infected pregnant women: ethical considerations. Am J Obstet Gynecol 1990;163:1111-4.

Minkoff H, Nanda D, Menes R, Fikrig S. Pregnancies resulting in infants with acquired immunodeficiency syndrome or AIDS-related complex: follow-up of mothers, children, and subsequently born siblings. Obstet Gynecol 1987;(69):288-91.

Mintz M. Neurologic abnormalities. In: Yogev, R, Connor EM, editors. Management of HIV infection in infants and children. St. Louis: Mosby Year Book; 1992. p. 247-85.

Mintz M, Epstein LG. Neurologic manifestations of pediatric acquired immunodeficiency syndrome: clinical features and therapeutic approaches. Semin Neurol 1992;12:51-6.

Mintz M, Epstein LG, Koenigsberger MR. Neurological manifestations of acquired immunodeficiency syndrome in children. Int Pediatr 1989;4(2):161-71.

Mintz M, Rapaport R, Oleske J et al. Elevated serum levels of tumor necrosis factors are associated with progressive encephalopathy in children with acquired immunodeficiency syndrome. Am J Dis Child 1989 Jun;143:771-4.

Monforte A, Novati R, Galli M et al. T-cell subsets and serum immunoglobulin levels in infants born to HIV-seropositive mothers: a longitudinal evaluation. AIDS 1990;4(11):1141-4.

Montgomery WP, Young RC, Allen MP, Harden KA. The tuberculin test in pregnancy. Am J Obstet Gynecol 1968;100(6):829-31.

Moore RD, Hidalgo J, Sugland BW, Chaisson RE. Zidovudine and the natural history of the acquired immunodeficiency syndrome. N Engl J Med 1991;324(20):1412-6.

Moore RD, Keruly J, Richman DD et al. Natural history of advanced HIV disease in patients treated with zidovudine. AIDS 1992;6(7):671-7.

Moore S. Case management and the integration of services: how service delivery systems shape case management. Soc Work 1992;37(5):418-23.

Mor V, Piette J, Fleishman J. Community-based case management for persons with AIDS. Health Aff (Millwood) 1989 Winter;8(4):139-53.

Moreno S, Baraia-Etxaburu J, Bouza E et al. Risk for developing tuberculosis among anergic patients infected with HIV. Ann Intern Med 1993 Aug;119(3):194-8.

Murray JF, Garay SM, Hopewell PC et al. NHLBI workshop summary: pulmonary complications of the acquired immunodeficiency syndrome. Am Rev Resp Dis 1987;135:504-8.

Musher DM, Hamill RJ, Baughn RE. Effect of human immunodeficiency virus (HIV) infection on the course of syphilis and on the response to treatment. Ann Intern Med 1990;113(11):872-81.

Nadal D, Hunziker UA, Schüpbach J et al. Immunological evaluation in the early diagnosis of prenatal or perinatal HIV infection. Arch Dis Child 1989 May;64(5):662-9.

National Center for Health Statistics. Advance report of final mortality statistics 1989. Monthly Vital Stat Rep 1992 Jan;40:1-52.

National Commission on AIDS. America living with AIDS. Washington: Author; 1991.

National Commission on AIDS. AIDS: an expanding tragedy. The final report of the National Commission on AIDS. Washington: Author; 1993.

National Institute of Allergy and Infectious Diseases. NIAID AIDS Research. Fiscal year 1991 report. Bethesda, MD: Author; 1991.

National Institute of Allergy and Infectious Diseases. News from NIAID: The effectiveness of AZT alone, ddC alone or AZT/ddC combination is similar overall for patients with advanced HIV disease. Bethesda, MD: Author; 1993a Jun;1-4.

National Institute of Allergy and Infectious Diseases. News from NIAID: ddI and ddC show similar benefits in advanced HIV disease: new options for people who cannot take or who no longer benefit from AZT. Bethesda, MD: Author; 1993b Jan 22;1-4.

National Institute of Allergy and Infectious Diseases. Community programs for clinical research on AIDS. Preliminary results of NIAID/CPCRA study 008, tuberculosis. Booster study. Bethesda, MD:Author; 1993c.

National Institutes of Health. State of the art conference on azidothymidine therapy of early HIV infection. Am J Med 1990; 89:335-344.

National Institutes of Health. NIH/ADAMHA policy concerning inclusion of women in study populations. NIH guide for grants and contracts; Oct 1986. NIH guide for grants and contracts (revised); 1991 Feb;20(3).

National Institutes of Health. Revitalization act of 1993. Public Law 103-43; 1993 Jun 10.

National Pediatric HIV Resource Center. Getting a head start on HIV. A resource manual for enhancing services to HIV-affected children in Head Start. Newark, NJ; Author; 199a. p. 1-56.

National Pediatric HIV Resource Center. Antiretroviral therapy and medical management of HIV-infected children. Pediatr Infect Dis J 1993;12:513-22.

New York City Department of Health. Congenital syphilis: its prevention and control. City Health Information 1989;8:1-4.

Nix C, Cabaj P. Case management for substance abusers. Focus: a guide to AIDS research and counseling 1992 Sep;7(10):5-6.

Nolan K. Human immunodeficiency virus infection, women and pregnancy: ethical issues. Obstet Gynecol Clin N Am 1990;17:651-68.

Noronha D, Pallangyo KJ, Ndosi BN et al. Radiological features of pulmonary tuberculosis in patients infected with human immunodeficiency virus. East Afr Med J 1991;68(3):210-5.

Northfelt DW, Clement MJ, Safrin S. Extrapulmonary pneumocystosis: clinical features in human immunodeficiency virus infection. Medicine 1990;69(6):392-8.

Novello A. HIV in adolescence. Report of the Surgeon General's Task Force on HIV in Children and Adolescents and Families. Washington: Department of Health and Human Services; 1993.

Novello AC, Allen JR. Family-centered comprehensive care for children with HIV infection. Washington: Department of Health and Human Services); 1991.

Odeh M. The role of tumor necrosis factor-alpha in acquired immunodeficiency syndrome. J Intern Med 1990;228(1):549-56.

O'Dell V. Fear of rejection: patients' reluctance to disclose HIV diagnoses [letter]. AIDS 1988 Dec;2(6):484-5.

Oleske JM. Natural history of HIV infection in children. Report of Surgeon General's Workshop on Children with HIV Infection and their Families. Washington: Department of Health and Human Services (US); 1987. p. 24-5.

Oleske JM, McSherry GD, Altman R et al. Identification and initial management of HIV-infected infants and children in New Jersey. A practical protocol for New Jersey clinicians. The Academy of Medicine, Lawrenceville NJ, and New Jersey State Department of Health, Trenton, NJ; 1992. p. 52.

O'Sullivan MJ, Boyer P, Scott G et al. A phase 1 study of the pharmacokinetics and safety of zidovudine in third trimester HIV-1 infected pregnant women and their infants. Pediatr Res 1992 Apr;31(4):173A.

Owens DK, Nease RF. Development of outcome-based practice guidelines: a method for structuring problems and synthesizing evidence. Joint Commission J Qual Improve 1993; 19:248-63.

Oxtoby MJ. Human immunodeficiency virus and other viruses in human milk: placing the issues in a broader perspective. Pediatr Infect Dis J 1988;7:825-35.

Oxtoby MJ. Perinatally acquired human immunodeficiency virus infection. Pediatr Infect Dis J 1990;9:609-19.

Pahwa S, Chirmule N, Leombruno C et al. In vitro synthesis of human immunodeficiency virus-specific antibodies in peripheral blood lymphocytes in infants. Proc Natl Acad Sci USA 1989;86(5):7532-6.

Palumbo P, Jandinski J, Connor EM et al. Medical management of children with HIV infection. Pediatr Dent 1990;12:139-42.

Park YD, Belman AL, Kim T-S et al. Stroke in pediatric acquired immunodeficiency syndrome. Ann Neurol 1990 Sep;28(3):303-11.

Parker WA. Heterogeneity of the epitopes of CD4+ in patients infected with HIV. N Engl J Med 1988;319:581-2.

Parry GJ. Peripheral neuropathies associated with human immunodeficiency virus infection. Ann Neurol 1988;23(Suppl):S49-53.

Pazen GJ. Counseling must precede testing for HIV/AIDS. Penn Med 1991 Apr;94(4):22, 24-5.

Phelan JA, Eisig S, Freedman PD et al. Major aphthous-like ulcers in patients with AIDS. Oral Surg Oral Med Oral Pathol 1991;71:68-72.

Physician Payment Review Commission. Annual Report to Congress, 1993. Washington: Author; 1993.

Piette J, Fleishman J, Mor V, Thompson B. The structure and process of AIDS case management. Health Soc Work 1992 Feb;17(1):47-56.

Pincus-Strom D. Developing comprehensive services for HIV infected intravenous drug users: a guide for case managers [abstract M.E.P.62]. Int Conf AIDS. 1989 Jun 4-9; Montreal. p. S844.

Pindborg JJ. Classification of oral lesions associated with HIV infection. Oral Surg Oral Med Oral Pathol 1989;67:292-5.

Pitchenik AE, Rubinson HA. The radiographic appearance of tuberculosis in patients with the acquired immune deficiency syndrome (AIDS) and pre-AIDS. Am Rev Respir Dis 1985;131(3):393-6.

Pizzo P. Considerations for the evaluation of antiretroviral agents in infants and children infected with human immunodeficiency virus: a perspective from the National Cancer Institute. Rev Infect Dis 1990 Jul-Aug;12(Suppl 5):S561-9.

Pizzo PA, Butler K, Balis F et al. Dideoxycytidine alone and in an alternating schedule with AZT in children with symptomatic HIV infection. J Pediatr 1990 Nov; 117(5):799-808.

Pizzo PA, Eddy J, Falloon J et al. Effect of continuous intravenous infusion of zidovudine (AZT) in children with symptomatic HIV infection. N Engl J Med 1988;319(14):889-96.

Polk BF. Predictors of the acquired human immunodeficiency syndrome developing in a cohort of seropositive homosexual men. N Engl J Med 1987;158:615-22.

Present PA, Comstock GW. Tuberculin sensitivity in pregnancy. Am Rev Resp Dis 1975;112:413-6.

Preventive Services Task Force (US). Guide to clinical preventive services. An assessment of the effectiveness of 169 interventions. Baltimore: Williams & Wilkins; 1989.

Price DB, Inglese CM, Jacobs J et al. Pediatric AIDS: neuroradiologic and neurodevelopmental findings. Pediatr Radiol 1988;18:445-8.

Price RW, Brew B, Sidtis J et al. The brain in AIDS: central nervous system HIV-1 infection and AIDS dementia complex. Science 1988;239, 586-92.

Provencher D, Valme B, Avarette HE et al. HIV status and positive Papanicolaou screening: identification of a high-risk population. Gynecol Oncol 1988;31:184-8.

Quinn TC, Cannon RD, Glasser D. The association of syphilis with risk of human immunodeficiency virus infection in patients attending sexually transmitted disease clinics. Arch Intern Med 1990;150(6):1297-302.

Quinn TC, Kline R, Halsey N et al. Early diagnosis of perinatal HIV infection by detection of viral-specific IgA antibodies. JAMA 1991 Dec;226(24):3439-42.

Radolf JD, Kaplan RP. Unusual manifestations of secondary syphilis and abnormal humeral response to Treponema pallidum antigens in a homosexual man with asymptomatic human immunodeficiency virus infection. J Am Acad Dermatol 1988;18(Suppl 2):423-8.

Reamer FG. Aids, social work, and the "duty to protect." Soc Work 1991 Jan;36(1):56-60.

Rekart ML, Knowles L, Spencer D, Pengelly B. Patient referral or provider referral partner notification: which do patients prefer? [abstract S.C.103]. Int Conf AIDS; 1990 Jun 20-23. p. 121.

Rellihan MA, Dooley DP, Burke TW et al. Rapidly progressing cervical cancer in a patient with human immunodeficiency virus infection. Gynecol Oncol 1990;36(3):435-8.

Richman DD. Effect of stage of disease and drug dose on zidovudine susceptibilities of isolates of human immunodeficiency virus. J Acquir Immune Defic Syndr 1990;3(8):743-6.

Robert Wood Johnson Foundation. Weisfeld V, editor. AIDS health services at the crossroads: lessons for community care. Princeton, NJ: Author. 1991.

Robert CF, Hirschel B, Rochat T, Deglon JJ. Tuberculin skin reactivity in HIV-seropositive intravenous drug addicts [letter, comments]. N Engl J Med 1989;321(18):1268.

Rogers MF, Ou C-Y, Rayfield M et al. Use of the polymerase chain reaction for early detection of the proviral sequences of human immunodeficiency virus in infants born to seropositive mothers. N Engl J Med 1989;320:1649-54.

Rosenblum ML, Levy RM, Bredesen DE. AIDS and the nervous system. New York: Raven Press; 1988.

Rotheram-Borus MJ, Koopman C, Haignere C, Davies M. Reducing HIV sexual risk behaviors among runaway adolescents. JAMA 1991;266(9):1237-41.

Rounds KA. AIDS in rural areas: challenges to providing care. Soc Work 1988 May/Jun;33(3):257-61.

Royce RA, Luckman RS, Fusaro RE, Winkelstein W. The natural history of HIV-1 infection: staging classifications of disease. AIDS 1991;5:255-364.

Rudin C, Senn HP, Berger R et al. Repeated polymerase chain reaction complementary to other conventional methods for early detection of HIV infection in infants born to HIV-infected mothers. Eur J Clin Microbiol Infect Dis 1991;10:146-56.

Ruskin J, LaRiviere M. Low dose co-trimoxazole for prevention of Pneumocystis carinii pneumonia in human immunodeficiency virus disease [see comments]. Lancet 1991 Feb 23;337(8739):468-71.

Rutstein R. Predicting risk of Pneumocystis carinii pneumonia in human immunodeficiency virus-infected children. Am J Dis Child 1991 Aug;145(8):922-4.

Ryder RW, Nsa W, Hassig SE et al. Perinatal transmission of human immunodeficiency virus type-1 to infants of seropositive women in Zaire. N Engl J Med 1989 Jun;320(25):1637-42.

Saad MH, Kritski AL, Werneck EB, Fonseca LS. Use of the mycobacterial antigens for the serodiagnosis of tuberculosis in HIV-positive and HIV-negative individuals. World Conference on Lung Health; Boston; 1990 May 20-24. Am Rev Respir Dis 1990;141(4 part 2):A266.

Sande MA, Carpenter CCJ, Cobbs et al. Antiretroviral therapy for adult HIV-infected patients. JAMA 1993; 270(21):2583-9.

Schäfer A, Friedmann W, Mielke M et al. The increased frequency of cervical dysplasia-neoplasia in women infected with the human immunodeficiency virus is related to the degree of immunosuppression. Am J Obstet Gynecol 1991;164(2):593-9.

Scheinhorn DJ, Angelillo VA. Antituberculous therapy in pregnancy: risks to the fetus. West J Med 1977;127(3):195-8.

Schneider MME, Hoepelman AIM, Schattenkerk JKME et al. A controlled trial of aerosolized pentamidine or trimethoprim-sulfamethoxazole as primary prophylaxis against Pneumocystis carinii pneumonia in patients with human immunodeficiency virus infection. N Engl J Med 1992;327:1836-41.

Schott V. AIDS: a case for case management. Admit Manage J 1988 Fall;14(2):13-4.

Schrager LK, Friedland GH, Maude D et al. Cervical and vaginal squamous cell abnormalities in women infected with human immunodeficiency virus. J Acquir Immune Defic Syndr 1989;2(6):570-5.

Schulten EAJM, Reinier W, Van der Waal I. The impact of oral examination on the Centers for Disease Control classification of subjects with human immunodeficiency virus infection. Arch Intern Med 1990;1259-61.

Schuster GS, Schuster G. Oral microbiology and infectious diseases. 3rd ed. Philadelphia: BC Decker, Inc.; 1990.

Scott GB, Hutto C, Makuch RW et al. Survival in children with perinatally acquired human immunodeficiency virus type 1 infection. N Engl J Med 1989 Dec;321(26):1791-6.

Scully C, Laskaris G, Pindborg J et al. Oral manifestations of HIV infection and their management. I. More common lesions. Oral Surg Oral Med Oral Pathol 1991;71:158-66.

Selwyn PA, Alcabes P, Hartel D et al. Clinical manifestations and predictors of disease progression in a cohort of HIV-infected drug injectors. N Engl J Med 1992;326(24):1697-703.

Selwyn PA, Carter RJ, Schoenbaum EE et al. Knowledge of HIV antibody status and decisions to continue or terminate pregnancy among intravenous drug users. JAMA 1989 Jun;261(24):3567-71.

Selwyn PA, Hartel D, Lewis VA et al. A prospective study of the risk of tuberculosis among intravenous drug users with human immunodeficiency virus infection. N Engl J Med 1989;320(9):545-50.

Semprini AE, Ravizza M, Bucceri A et al. Perinatal outcome in HIV-infected pregnant women. Gynecol Obstet Invest 1990;30(1):15-8.

Sharer LR, Dowling PC, Michaels J et al. Spinal cord disease in children with HIV-1 infection: a combined molecular, biological and neuropathological study. Neuropathol Appl Neurobiol 1990;16:317-31.

Sharer LR, Epstein LG, Cho E-S et al. Pathologic features of AIDS encephalopathy in children: evidence for LAV/HTLV-lll infection of the brain. Hum Pathol 1986;17(3):271-84.

Sharer LR, Mintz M. The neuropathology of AIDS in children. In: Scaravilli F, editor. AIDS: the pathology of the nervous system. Berlin: Springer Verlag; in press.

Shaw GM, Hahn BH, Epstein LG et al. HTLV-III infection in brains of children and adults with AIDS encephalopathy. Science 1985;277:177-81.

Sheiham A. Is there a scientific basis for six monthly dental examinations? Lancet 1977;2:442-4.

Shiboski CH, Greenspan D, Westenhouse JL et al. Prevalence of oral lesions in a cohort of HIV-seropositive women. J Dent Res 1992;71:172.

Shulman LC, Mantell JE. The AIDS crisis: a United States health care perspective. Soc Sci Med 1988;26:979-88.

Siena Conference. Maternal factors involved in mother-to-child transmission of HIV-1. J Acquir Immune Defic Syndr 1992;5:1019-29.

Sierra Health Foundation. Challenges for the future: coordinating HIV/AIDS care and services in the next decade. Report of National Symposium on Case Management and HIV/AIDS; 1992. p. 1-37.

Sillman F, Stanek A, Sedlis A et al. The relationship between human papilloma virus and lower genital intraepithelial neoplasia in immunosuppressed women. Am J Obstet Gynecol 1984;150(3):300-8.

Simpson DM. Neuromuscular complications of human immunodeficiency virus infection. Semin Neurol 1992;12:34-42.

Smith GM, Forbes MA, Cooper J et al. Prognostic indicators for the development of AIDS in HIV antibody positive haemophiliac patients: results of a three year longitudinal study. Clin Lab Haematol 1991;13:115-25.

Snider DE. The tuberculin skin test. Am Rev Resp Dis 1982;125(3, pt 2):108-18.

Snider DE, Layde PM, Johnson MW, Lyle MA. Treatment of tuberculosis during pregnancy. Am Rev Resp Dis 1980;122:65-79.

Sonenstein FL, Pleck JH, Ku LC. Sexual activity, condom use and AIDS awareness among adolescent males. Fam Plann Perspect 1989;21(4):152-8.

Sonsel GE, Paradise F, Stroup S. Case management practice in an AIDS service organization. Soc Casework 1988 Jun;69(6):388-92.

Sperling R, Stratton P, O'Sullivan MJ et al. A survey of zidovudine use in pregnant women with human immunodeficiency virus infection. N Engl J Med 1992;326:857-61.

St Louis ME, Conway GA, Hayman CR et al. Human immunodeficiency virus infection in disadvantaged adolescents. JAMA 1991;266(17):2387-91.

Stafl A, Mattingly RF. Colposcopic diagnosis of cervical neoplasia. Obstet Gynecol 1973;41:168.

Stein DS, Korvick JA, Vermund SM. CD4 lymphocyte cell enumeration for prediction of clinical course of human immunodeficiency virus disease: a review. J Infect Dis 1992;165(2):352-63.

Stein J, Roche N, Mathur-Wagh U et al. Gynecologic findings in an HIV positive outpatient population (abstract M.B. 2427). Int Conf AIDS; 1991. p. 129

Stricof RL. HIV seroprevalence in a facility for runaway and homeless adolescents. Am J Public Health 1991;50:232-6.

Sunderam G, McDonald RJ, Maniatis T et al. Tuberculosis as a manifestation of the acquired immunodeficiency syndrome (AIDS). JAMA 1986;256(3):362-6.

Svensson CK. Representation of American blacks in clinical trials of new drugs. JAMA 1989;261:2709-12.

Swango PA, Kleinman DV, Konzelman JL. HIV and periodontal health. J Am Dent Assoc 1992;122:49-54.

Swartz HM, Reichling BA. Hazards of radiation exposure for pregnant women. JAMA 1978;239(18):1907-8.

Tanner JM. Growth at adolescence: with a general consideration of the effects of hereditary and environmental factors upon growth and maturation from birth to maturity. 2nd ed. Oxford: Blackwell Scientific Publications; 1962. 325 p.

Tasker M. How can I tell you? Secrecy and disclosure with children when a family member has AIDS. Bethesda (MD): Association for Care of Children's Health; 1992 Feb.

Telzak EE, Greenberg MSZ, Harrison J et al. Syphilis treatment response in infected individuals. AIDS 1991;5:591-5.

Temmerman M, Plummer FA, Mirza NB et al. Infection with HIV as a risk factor for adverse obstetrical outcome. AIDS 1990 Nov;4(11):1087-93.

Tenenbaum HC, Mock D, Simor AE. Periodontitis as an early presentation of HIV infection. Can Med Assoc J 1991;144:1265-9.

Thomas P, Lubin K, Milberg J et al. Cohort comparison study of children whose mothers have acquired immunodeficiency syndrome and children of well inner city mothers. Pediatr Infect Dis J 1987 Mar;6(3):247-51.

Tikjob G, Russel M, Petersen CS et al. Seronegative secondary syphilis in a patient with AIDS: Identification of Treponema pallidum in biopsy specimen [brief commentary]. J Am Acad Dermatol 1991;24:506-8.

Tollerud DJ, Ildstad ST, Brown LM et al. T-cell subsets in healthy teenagers: transition to the adult phenotype. Clin Immunol Immunopathol 1990 Jul;55-56(1):88-96.

Toomey KE, Cates W Jr. Partner notification for the prevention of HIV infection. AIDS 1989;3(Suppl 1):S57-62.

Townsend DE, Ostergard DR, Mishell DR, Hirose SM. Abnormal Papanicolaou smears: evaluation by colposcopy, biopsies and endocervical curettage. Am J Obstet Gynecol 1970;108:429.

Tramont EC. Treponema pallidum (syphilis). In: Mandell GL, Douglas RG Jr, Bennett JE, editors. Principles and practice of infectious disease. 5th ed. New York: Churchill Livingston; 1990. p. 1794-808.

Tudor-Williams G, St Clair MH, McKinney RE et al. HIV-1 sensitivity to zidovudine and clinical outcome in children. Lancet 1992;339:15-9.

Tukutuku K, Muyembe-Tramfun L, Kayembe K, Ntumba M. Oral manifestations of AIDS in a heterosexual population in a Zaire hospital. J Pathol Med 1990;19:232-4.

Tuset C, Elorza JF, Tuset L et al. The utility of a number of AIDS evaluation markers in the follow-up of the vertical transmission of HIV infection [abstract F.B.433]. Int Conf AIDS. 1990 Jun 20-23. p. 188.

Ujhelyi E, Fuchs D, Králl G et al. Age dependency of the progression of HIV disease in haemophiliacs: predictive value of T-cell subsets and neopterin measurements. Immunol Lett 1990;26(1):67-74.

Vermund SH, Kelley KF, Klein RS et al. High risk of human papillomavirus infection and cervical squamous intraepithelial lesions among women with symptomatic human immunodeficiency virus infection. Am J Obstet Gynecol 1991;165(2):392-400.

Vernon DD, Holzman BH, Lewis P et al. Respiratory failure in children with acquired immunodeficiency syndrome-related complex. Pediatrics 1988;82:223-8.

Volberding PA, Lagakos SW, Koch MA et al. Zidovudine in asymptomatic human immunodeficiency virus infection. A controlled trial in persons with fewer than 500 CD4-positive cells per cubic millimeter. The AIDS Clinical Trials Group of the National Institute of Allergy and Infectious Diseases [see comments]. N Engl J Med 1990;322(14):941-9.

Walter EB, Drucker RP, McKinney RE, Wilfert CM. Myopathy in human immunodeficiency virus-infected children receiving long term zidovudine therapy. Pediatrics 1991;90:152-5.

Warkany J. Antituberculous drugs. Teratology 1979;20:133-8.

Watts DH, Brown ZA, Tartaglione T. Pharmacokinetic disposition of zidovudine during pregnancy. J Infect Dis 1991;163:226-32.

Weiblen BJ, Lee FK, Cooper ER et al. Early diagnoses of HIV infection in infants by detection of IgA HIV antibodies. Lancet 1990;335(8696):988-90.

Weinstein L, Murphy T. The management of tuberculosis during pregnancy. Clin Perinatol 1974;1:395.

Werhane MJ, Torbeck GS, Schrufnagel DE. The tuberculosis clinic. Chest 1991;96(4):815-8.

White MV, Haddad ZH, Brunner E, Sainz C. Desensitization to trimethoprim sulfamethoxazole in patients with acquired immune deficiency syndrome and Pneumocystis carinii pneumonia. Ann Allergy 1989;62:177-9.

Wilson LB, Coover MO. Case management: review of national best practice models. Dallas: University of Texas Health Science Center; 1985.

Winkler JR, Murray PA, Grassi M, Hammerle C. Diagnosis and management of HIV-associated periodontal lesions. J Am Dent Assoc 1989; 119(Suppl):S25-34.

Wolters P, Brouwers P, Moss H. The effect of 2', 3' dideoxysine (ddI) on the cognitive functioning of infants and children with symptomatic HIV infection [abstract S.B.205]. Int Conf AIDS; 1990 Jun 20-23.

World Health Organization (WHO). Global Programme on AIDS: current and future dimensions of the HIV/AIDS pandemic. A capsule summary. Geneva: WHO; 1992 Jan.

Worth D. Sexual decision making and AIDS: why condom promotion among vulnerable women is likely to fail. Stud Fam Plann 1989;6:297-307.

Wright T. Columbia University, New York, NY. Personal communication. 1993.

Zeballos RS, Cavalcante N, Freire CA, et al. Intracutaneous tests with ubiquitous antigens and CD4-CD8 determinations in AIDS [abstract B.369]. Int Conf AIDS; 1989 Jun 4-9. p. 504.

Acronyms

AGOG	American College of Obstetricians and Gynecologists
ACTG	AIDS Clinical Trials Group
AFB	acid-fast bacillus
AHCPR	Agency for Health Care Policy and Research
AIDS	acquired immunodeficiency syndrome
AZT	azidothymidine
BCG	bacille Calmette-Guerin
CDC	Centers for Disease Control and Prevention
CIN	cervical intraepithelial neoplasia
CMV	cytomegalovirus
CNS	central nervous system
CPCRA	Community Programs for Clinical Research on AIDS
CSF	cerebrospinal fluid
CT	computerized tomographic [scan]
ddC	2', 3'-dideoxycytidine (zalcitabine)
ddI	2', 3'-dideoxyinosine (didanosine)
DFA-TP	direct fluorescent antibody staining for *Treponema pallidum*
DOT	directly observed therapy
ELISA	enzyme-linked immunosorbent assay
FDA	Food and Drug Administration
FTA-ABS	fluorescent treponemal antibody absorption
G6PD	glucose-6-phosphate dehydrogenase
HIV	human immunodeficiency virus
HPV	human papilloma virus
IFA	immunofluorescence antibody
IgG	immunoglobulin G
IM	intramuscular
IND	investigational new drug

INH	isoniazid
IV	intravenous
LIP	lymphoid interstitial pneumonitis
LP	lumbar puncture
MACS	Multicenter AIDS Cohort Study
MDR-TB	multidrug-resistant tuberculosis
MHA-TP	microhemagglutination assay for *Treponema pallidum*
MRI	magnetic resonance imaging
NIAID	National Institute of Allergy and Infectious Diseases
NICHD	National Institute of Child Health and Human Development
NIH	National Institutes of Health
NLM	National Library of Medicine
OI	opportunistic infection
Pap	Papanicolaou [smear]
PCP	*Pneumocystis carinii* pneumonia
PCR	polymerase chain reaction
PPD	purified protein derivative
RPR	rapid plasma reagin
SIL	squamous intraepithelial lesion
STD	sexually transmitted disease
TB	tuberculosis
TMP-SMX	trimethoprim-sulfamethoxazole
TU	tuberculin unit
VDRL	Venereal Disease Research Laboratories
WHO	World Health Organization
ZDV	zidovudine

Glossary

Access: The degree of ease with which the consumer can secure health services. Along with availability, access is a key criterion used to measure the adequacy of a health care system.

Acid-fast bacillus (AFB): Any bacillus that is resistant to decolorization with acidified organic solvents after staining with a dye. Used as the basis of a test for identifying *Mycobacterium tuberculosis* and other mycobacteria.

Acquired immunodeficiency syndrome (AIDS): A manifestation of infection with the human immunodeficiency virus (HIV) characterized by the presence of one or more diseases as defined by the Centers for Disease Control and Prevention (CDC). These diseases occur following a depression of an individual's immune system function. The affected person becomes susceptible to unusual infections and malignancies (see "opportunistic infection").

Adherence: The act of following a prescribed therapeutic regimen.

Advocacy: Action taken on behalf of individuals by themselves, their families, health care providers, or others to ensure appropriate access to and availability of health care services.

Aerosolized pentamidine: A drug used for *Pneumocystis carinii* pneumonia (PCP) prophylaxis that is dispersed through a nebulizer in a mist. When inhaled, it goes directly to the lungs.

AFB isolation: A specific type of hospital isolation for persons with acute *M. tuberculosis*. Its purpose is to prevent the spread of infection during the infectious phase of the disease.

Agency for Health Care Policy and Research (AHCPR): Agency within the Public Health Service, U.S. Department of Health and Human Services, that sponsors research on the effectiveness and cost-effectiveness of medical care.

AIDS Clinical Trials Group (ACTG): Project under which 50 medical centers nationwide are participating in the evaluation of treatments for HIV-related infections. Sponsored by the National Institute of Allergy and Infectious Diseases.

Airborne transmission: Process by which an infectious agent passes through the air to infect susceptible individuals by droplet infection (e.g., sneezing, coughing).

Americans with Disabilities Act: (Public Law 101-336) Passed in July 1990, this legislation establishes equal opportunity for persons with disabilities regarding employment, public accommodation, transportation, State and local government services, and telecommunications.

Anergy: State of being unable to react immunologically to an antigenic stimulus. Usually used to denote lack of response to specific antigens injected into the skin of the forearm.

Antibodies: Proteins in the blood or secretory fluids that tag and help remove or neutralize bacteria, viruses, and other harmful toxins. Antibodies are members of a class of proteins known as immunoglobulins, which are produced and secreted by B-lymphocytes in response to stimulation by antigens.

Antigen: Any foreign substance that evokes an immune response when introduced into the body.

Antiretroviral drug: A drug that reduces the replication rate of HIV and is used to treat HIV-infected persons. The most commonly used are zidovudine, didanosine, and zalcitabine.

Aphthous ulcers: Single or multiple recurrent, well-circumscribed painful ulcers that develop on nonkeratinized oral mucosa.

Asymptomatic HIV infection: An early stage of HIV infection in which the patient has no physical symptoms.

Atypical cells of undetermined significance (ACUS): Abnormal cells with certain characteristics that are revealed on Pap smear.

Availability: Term used in describing the degree to which health care services, including facilities and personnel, are in place and readily accessible to all consumers.

Azidothymidine (AZT): 3'-azido-2', 3'-dideoxythymidine (see zidovudine).

Bacille Calmette-Guerin (BCG): A vaccine containing a bovine-derived, live, attenuated strain of mycobacterium that has been used in countries other than the United States as immunization against tuberculosis.

Beta-2-microglobulin (B2M): A protein that is tightly bound to the surface of all cells with a nucleus. B2M is released into the blood when a cell dies. Elevated B2M levels occur in a variety of diseases and cancers. Although B2M is nonspecific for HIV infection, there is a correlation between elevated B2M levels and progression of HIV disease.

Body fluids: The various liquids found in the human body. Of these fluids, only blood, semen, vaginal secretions, and breast milk have been found to contain concentrations of HIV that are high enough to infect another person. Saliva, sweat, tears, and urine have not been shown to transmit HIV.

Bronchoscopy: Visualization of the trachea and lungs with a flexible fiberoptic tube.

CD4 cell count (T4 count): The most characterized of all the surrogate markers of immunodeficiency; the number of CD4 (T4 helper) cells. As an HIV-infected individual's CD4 cells decline, the risk of developing opportunistic infections increases. The trend of several consecutive CD4 counts is more important than any one measurement.

Candidiasis: An infection with a fungus of the *Candida* family, generally *C. albicans,* that most commonly involves the skin (dermatocandidiasis), oral mucosa (thrush), respiratory tract (bronchocandidiasis), and vagina (vaginitis). Candidiasis of the esophagus, trachea, bronchi, or lungs is an indicator disease for AIDS.

Carcinoma in situ: An early, curable stage of cancer in which the tumor has not spread beyond a defined superficial site.

Case management: System under which the patient's health care and social services are coordinated by one or more individuals familiar with both the patient's needs and community resources.

Casual contact: In the context of AIDS, refers to nonintimate behaviors such as working, eating, playing, studying, hugging, or holding hands. These activities do not transmit HIV.

CD4 percentage: The number of CD4 cells in relation to the total number of lymphocytes. As HIV infection progresses, the percentage of CD4 cells decreases.

Centers for Disease Control and Prevention (CDC): Federal agency that is responsible for monitoring the AIDS/HIV epidemic and carrying out efforts to prevent HIV infection.

Central nervous system (CNS): The brain, spinal cord, and its coverings (meninges).

Cervical dysplasia: An abnormality in the size, shape, or organization of the cells lining the cervix that can be detected on a Pap smear. If undetected, cervical dysplasia may progress to a more severe lesion; thus, any abnormal finding should prompt further examination.

Cervical intraepithelial lesion (CIN): A condition revealed by Pap smear that necessitates further evaluation.

Childbearing age: The period of a woman's life during which she is capable of conceiving.

Client oriented: Describes medical and social services that are directed toward the client's or patient's needs and interests.

Clinical trials: Scientifically governed investigations of medications in volunteer subjects. Their purpose is to seek information regarding the products' safety (Phase I) and efficacy (Phase II/III).

Cohort: A group of individuals sharing a demographic or clinical characteristic.

Colposcopy: A procedure in which the surface of the uterine cervix is examined through a flexible fiberoptic tube.

Community based: Describes services delivered at a local level or as close to the client's home as possible.

Community Programs for Clinical Research on AIDS (CPCRA): A program involving 17 centers that conduct clinical trials related to HIV in community-based settings. Sponsored by the National Institute of Allergy and Infectious Diseases.

Comprehensive care: Care that includes the full spectrum of health, educational, social, and related services.

Condom: A sheath used to cover the penis during sexual intercourse to prevent conception and sexually transmitted diseases. Correct use of a rubber (latex) condom during every act of intercourse greatly reduces, but does not eliminate, the risk of infection with HIV. Lambskin or "natural" condoms do not offer protection because they are too porous.

Confidentiality: The right inherent in the contract between the health care provider and patient that ensures that information on the patient's medical conditions will be released to a third party only after explicit permission is obtained from the patient or guardian.

Congregate living: Any one of a number of housing, shelter, or confinement environments in which a number of individuals live together.

Consumer: An individual who uses a product or service. In the health care setting, a more general term for "client" or "patient."

Continuous care: Describes care that is maintained without interruption despite changes in site, caregiver, or method of payment.

Coordinated care: Describes care that is planned and implemented so as to form a cohesive therapeutic program.

Cotton-wool spots/patches: Fluffy-looking white deposits on the retina that represent small areas that have lost their blood supply due to blockage of local vessels.

Cytomegalovirus (CMV): A member of the herpes virus family that can cause fever, fatigue, enlarged lymph glands, aching, and mild sore throat. In persons with AIDS, CMV infections can produce hepatitis, pneumonia, retinitis, and colitis. CMV infection may lead to blindness, chronic diarrhea, or death.

Cytopenia: A reduction in the number of cells found in a clinical specimen.

Dapsone: A drug used for PCP prophylaxis; possible side effects include skin rash, fever, and gastrointestinal upset. In persons who have the hereditary condition glucose-6-phosphate dehydrogenase (G6PD) deficiency, dapsone can cause destruction of red blood cells (hemolysis).

Developmentally oriented: Describes care that is based on the individual's functional level and chronologic age. Functional level includes physical, cognitive, psychosocial, and communicative development.

Didanosine (ddI; trade name, Videx; also called dideoxyinosine): One of three nucleoside analog drugs currently approved by the Food and Drug Administration that inhibits the reverse transcriptase enzyme of HIV. Its major toxicities are pancreatitis and peripheral neuropathy.

Dideoxycytidine (ddC): 2', 3'-dideoxycytine; see zalcitabine.

Dideoxyinosine (ddI): 2', 3'-dideoxyinosine; see didanosine.

Direct fluorescent antibody staining for *Treponema pallidum* (DFA-TP): A specific test (direct fluorescent antibody staining on a biopsy sample) for *T. pallidum,* the organism that causes syphilis. The presence of *T. pallidum* organisms in lesions of early acquired or congenital syphilis in this test is the definitive means of making a diagnosis of syphilis.

Directly observed therapy (DOT): A process in which a patient takes a medication while under direct observation by another individual. Usually used in antituberculous treatment.

Double blind: A trial design in which neither the subjects nor the participating research investigators are aware of which patients are receiving test drugs and which are receiving placebo or other therapy. Believed to promote faster and more objective results, since it eliminates the possibility of bias concerning the test drug's efficacy.

Early HIV infection: The stage of HIV infection during which no major physical health symptoms are yet present, though psychological symptoms may be present.

Empiric therapy: Treatment based on the clinician's judgment and the patient's symptoms and signs and offered before a diagnosis has been confirmed.

Encephalopathy: Injury or damage to the brain.

Enzyme-linked immunosorbent assay (ELISA): The most common assay for HIV antibodies. Used for screening donated blood, it is usually the first clinical screening test used to detect HIV infection. A positive ELISA or EIA test result should be confirmed with a Western Blot or an immunofluorescent assay test in order to conclusively diagnose HIV infection.

Epidemic: An outbreak of contagious disease, such as HIV infection, that spreads rapidly within a population.

Expanded access: Refers to the concept of making experimental drugs more widely available to patients with life-threatening diseases prior to marketing approval. Information on the process is available through the FDA.

Family centered: Describes care that recognizes and respects the pivotal role of the family in the lives of children and other members. Supports families in their natural caregiving roles, promotes normal patterns of living, and ensures family collaboration and choice in the provision of services to members of the family who are sick.

Fluorescent treponemal antibody absorption test (FTA-ABS): A treponemal test to detect antibodies against *Treponema pallidum,* the organism that causes syphilis.

Food and Drug Administration (FDA): Federal agency responsible for approving new pharmaceutical products and medical devices and for monitoring drug performance following approval.

Funduscopy: Visual examination of the retina with an ophthalmoscope.

Glucose-6-phosphate dehydrogenase (G6PD) deficiency: An inherited enzyme deficiency that can lead to hemolysis of red blood cells (RBCs) when an affected individual is exposed to drugs with oxidant properties.

Guidelines: Clinical practice recommendations formulated by a consensus of experts or based on a literature review by a panel of experts and consumers. Purpose is to educate health care providers, improve the care provided to individuals with specified conditions, and, when possible, enhance the cost effectiveness of health care. Should be distinguished from "standards of care" in which providers are required to adhere to recommendations.

Hairy leukoplakia: A white lesion seen in the oral cavity of HIV-infected individuals, most commonly on the lateral margins of the tongue. It may be flat or raised with vertical corrugations and is not removable.

Health care facility: A freestanding edifice (licensed where required) dedicated to the provision of medical and nursing care.

Hemolysis: The destruction of red blood cells (RBCs) by the action of drugs, serum proteins (complement), infectious agents, or turbulent blood flow.

Hemoptysis: The coughing up of blood from the lungs; may be a symptom of tuberculosis.

HIV antibody (HIV-Ab): The antibody to HIV, which usually appears within 6 weeks after infection. Antibody testing early in the infection process may not produce accurate results, since some recently infected people have not yet begun producing antibodies and test negative even though they are infected. Thus, a single negative antibody test result is not a guarantee that a person is free from infection. The change from HIV-negative to HIV-positive status is called seroconversion.

HIV counseling: Information provided to an individual before and after HIV testing (pre- and posttest counseling) regarding the implications and impact of testing, HIV infection care, and prevention of HIV transmission.

HIV-infected: Infected with the human immunodeficiency virus, with or without evidence of illness.

HIV-negative: Not infected with HIV, as determined by a negative test for antibody to HIV or for the presence of the virus.

HIV-positive: Infected with HIV, as determined by a positive test for antibody to HIV or for the presence of the virus.

Home care: Medical care and related services that are given at home by family members, nurses or health care providers, or a combination thereof.

Hospice: A health facility in which medical and mental health care are provided to a terminally ill patient. The hospice philosophy emphasizes alleviating the patient's discomfort and supporting the family in the grieving process.

Human immunodeficiency virus (HIV): The organism isolated and recognized as the etiologic agent of AIDS. HIV is classified as a lentivirus in a subgroup of the retroviruses. It infects and destroys a class of lymphocytes, CD4 cells, thereby causing progressive damage to the immune system. This family of retroviruses has RNA as its genetic material and makes an enzyme, reverse transcriptase, that converts viral RNA into viral DNA. The viral DNA then is incorporated into the host cell's DNA and is replicated along with it. There are two known types of HIV: HIV-1 is the most common in the United States; HIV-2 causes a milder immune suppression and is found primarily in West Africa.

Human papilloma virus (HPV): The virus that causes genital warts. Certain types of HPV (types 16 and 18) are associated with cervical cancer.

Immunofluorescence antibody (IFA): A serologic assay using antibody tagged by a fluorescent molecule. There is an HIV-specific IFA assay available to confirm the results of a positive HIV ELISA test.

Immune system: The mechanism of the body that recognizes foreign agents or substances, neutralizes them, and recalls the response later when confronted with the same challenge.

Immunization: Administration of antigenic components of an infectious agent to stimulate a protective immune response.

Immunity: Natural or acquired resistance to a specific disease. Immunity may be partial or complete, long lasting or temporary.

Immunodeficiency: A breakdown or an inability of certain parts of the immune system to function that renders a person susceptible to certain diseases that he or she ordinarily would not develop.

Immunocompromised: Describes the condition that exists when the body's immune system defenses are lowered and the ability to resist infections and tumors weakens.

Immunoglobulin (Ig): Protein produced by plasma cells derived from B-lymphocytes and found in the blood and other body tissues. Increased levels of two types of immunoglobulins, IgA and IgG, are usually seen in patients with HIV infection and are related to the HIV-induced activation of B-lymphocytes. Immunoglobulin A is found in high concentrations in mucous membranes and in secretions such as saliva. It does not cross the placenta. Immunoglobulin G is found in the serum and does cross the placenta.

Incubation period: The interval between initial infection and appearance of the first symptom or sign of disease.

Informed consent: Process by which individuals considering participation in an investigational drug trial are informed by an investigator in simple terms of the risks and benefits of the proposed treatment and voluntarily agree to participate in the trial. The consent form is a written document that attests to the fact that the person signing understands the purposes and risks of the study. Also refers to the process in which an individual voluntarily consents to diagnostic testing and release of information (disclosure) after appropriate counseling.

Investigational new drug (IND): See Treatment IND.

In vitro: Testing and experiments conducted in a laboratory setting.

In vivo: Testing and experiments conducted in animals or humans.

Isoniazid (INH): An antibiotic that has activity against *M. tuberculosis,* the micro-organism that causes tuberculosis.

Kaposi's sarcoma (KS): A painless tumor of the wall of blood vessels or the lymphatic system that usually appears on the skin as pink-to-purple spots. It may also occur internally, independent of skin lesions.

Lumbar puncture (LP): Insertion of a needle into the spinal canal to obtain a sample of cerebrospinal fluid.

Lymphocyte: The most prominent cell type in the immune system. B-lymphocytes are one of the two major classes of lymphocytes. During infections, these cells are transformed into plasma cells that produce antibodies specific to the pathogen. This transformation occurs through interactions with various types of T-cells and other components of the immune system. T-lymphocytes are derived from the thymus and participate in a variety of cell-mediated immune reactions. Three fundamentally different types of T-cells are recognized: helper, killer, and suppressor.

Mandatory reporting: System under which a physician is required by law to inform health authorities when a specified illness is diagnosed. Mandatory reporting is required for AIDS in all 50 States, and it has been proposed that the requirement be extended to HIV infection.

Medicaid: Federal/State health care program for persons below the poverty level.

Medicare: Federal health insurance program for persons 65 years of age and older, the disabled, and those with end-stage renal disease.

Microhemagglutination assay for *T. pallidum* (MATP): A treponemal test for syphilis based on agglutination of red cells to which antigens from the micro-organism *T. pallidum* have been attached.

Multidrug-resistant tuberculosis (MDR-TB): Tuberculosis caused by a strain of the organism *Mycobacterium tuberculosis* that is resistant to more than one of the major antituberculous drugs.

***Mycobacterium avium-intracellular* complex (MAC):** An acid-fast micro-organism that causes lung and other organ system infections in individuals whose immune systems are severely damaged. Evidence of MAC has been found in approximately 50 percent of adult AIDS patients at autopsy.

Mycobacterium tuberculosis: The micro-organism that causes tuberculosis.

Myopathy: Inflammation of muscle tissue due to infection or adverse reaction to a medication.

National Institutes of Health (NIH): Agency of the Federal Government that funds and conducts biomedical research.

Neopterin: A molecule produced by macrophages in response to gamma interferon and found in serum, urine, and cerebrospinal fluid. Elevated neopterin levels have been reported in individuals in all phases of HIV disease. According to some studies, high neopterin levels have been associated with a poor prognosis; low levels have correlated with a better prognosis.

Neurodevelopmental delays: Changes in the level of functioning of the central nervous system that lead to the loss of skills that a child has developed or would have developed over time.

Neuropathy: An abnormal, degenerative, or inflammatory condition of the peripheral nervous system.

Neuropsychological defects: Alterations in behavior that are related to a central nervous system illness and interfere with an individual's ability to function in an age-appropriate fashion.

Neurosyphilis: A form of advanced syphilis in which the infection has spread to the central nervous system.

Nucleoside analog: A synthetic compound similar to one of the components of DNA or RNA; a general type of antiretroviral drug (e.g., acyclovir, zidovudine).

Nondirective counseling: Describes a type of counseling in which the counselor supplies information and helps the client to arrive at a decision that reflects the client's needs and wishes.

Opportunistic infections (OIs): Illnesses caused by organisms that do not usually cause disease in a person with a healthy immune system. When an individual's immune system is compromised, such organisms may cause serious, even life-threatening illness.

Optimal health: The highest state of well-being attainable by a person at a particular time in his or her life. Although the optimal health for an HIV-infected person may be different from that of someone who is HIV-negative, optimal health, defined in terms of the individual patient, should still be the goal for care of an HIV-infected individual.

Outreach worker: Professional or paraprofessional who actively seeks out patients in their own environments and communities and provides education and medical services.

p24 antigen test (p24 antigen capture assay): Laboratory test that measures p24, the protein found in the viral core of HIV. This test can sometimes detect HIV infection before seroconversion. p24 is consistently present in only about 25 percent of HIV-infected persons. Persistent p24 antigenemia has been associated with an increased risk of progression to AIDS in HIV-infected individuals.

Papanicolaou (Pap) smear: A microscopic examination of the surface cells of the cervix, usually conducted on scrapings from the opening of the cervix.

Pandemic: A disease occurring in epidemic proportions worldwide.

Parenteral: Intravenous or intramuscular administration of substances such as therapeutic drugs or nutritive solutions.

Partner notification: The process of informing sexual or needle-sharing partners of an HIV-infected person that they have been or are at risk of contracting HIV infection. May be done by the HIV-infected person, a health care provider, or a public health worker.

Pentamidine: A drug used for PCP prophylaxis and treatment.

Perinatal transmission: Transmission of HIV from mother to infant by blood or body fluids. May occur in utero, at the time of delivery, and possibly by breast-feeding.

Phase I clinical trial: Typically involves 20 to 100 patients and lasts several months. The major purpose is to determine safety and dose. Approximately 70 percent of drugs successfully complete phase I.

Phase II clinical trial: Typically involves up to several hundred patients and usually lasts from several months to 2 years. The major purposes are to continue to determine short-term safety and, primarily, effectiveness. Approximately 33 percent of drugs successfully complete phase II.

Phase III clinical trial: Typically involves from several hundred to several thousand patients and may last from 1 to 4 years. The major purposes are to study safety, effectiveness, and dosage. Approximately 25 to 30 percent of drugs successfully complete phase III.

***Pneumocystis carinii* pneumonia (PCP):** Form of pneumonia seen in persons with an impaired immune system, such as those who are HIV infected. PCP is the leading cause of death in patients with AIDS. It is caused by the opportunistic pathogen (unclear whether fungal or protozoan), *P. carinii,* which can infect the eyes, skin, spleen, liver, and heart, as well as the lungs.

Polymerase chain reaction (PCR): A laboratory technique employing molecular biology technology to identify the nucleic acid sequence of HIV in the cells of an infected individual. This technique is sensitive and can detect a single copy of viral DNA in 1 cell out of 10,000. It is useful for early detection of perinatally infected infants and monitoring patients on clinical trials.

Pregnancy counseling: Process of discussing with a woman of childbearing age her options regarding whether to become pregnant or, if she is already pregnant, whether to continue or terminate the pregnancy.

Primary care provider: A health care provider (e.g., physician, physician assistant, nurse practitioner) who offers and coordinates comprehensive patient care.

Primary care setting: A place where comprehensive care is delivered (e.g., a physician's office, community health clinic, preventive nursing service).

Prophylaxis: Intervention intended to preserve health and prevent the initial occurrence of a disease (primary prophylaxis) or to prevent the recurrence of a disease (secondary prophylaxis).

Prozone phenomenon: A reaction that occurs in undiluted or slightly diluted serum in which antibody is present in such high concentration that it interferes with precipitation reactions with antigens. The phenomenon may interfere with obtaining a correct result from a test, especially a test for syphilis.

Pruritus: The symptom of itching. It may be paroxysmal or constant and may be associated with skin lesions or occur independent of any skin lesion.

Purified protein derivative (PPD): Protein-rich material derived from the microorganism *M. tuberculosis* and used as a skin-test reagent to detect current or prior infection with that organism.

Pyrazinamide: An antibiotic used as part of multidrug combinations to treat tuberculosis.

Quality of life: Expression used in speaking of issues relating to normalizing the life of a chronically ill individual. In defining quality of life, health care providers must consider not only the physical responses to medical therapy, but also the psychological implications of illness for both the patient and family. The overriding goal of care should be to relieve suffering and increase patient well-being.

Randomized: Term used to describe a study in which participants in a drug trial randomly receive one of the treatments being studied or a placebo.

Rapid plasma reagin (RPR): A nontreponemal test for detection of syphilis, the basis of which is agglutination.

Retinitis: Inflammation of the retina; linked to cytomegalovirus infection in persons with AIDS. Untreated, it can cause blindness.

Risk reduction: Process by which an individual changes behavior so as to decrease the likelihood of acquiring an infection.

Ryan White CARE (Comprehensive AIDS Resources Emergency) Act: Passed in 1990 to provide services for persons with HIV infection, this act seeks "to improve the quality and availability of care for individuals and families with HIV disease." It directs financial assistance to metropolitan areas with the largest numbers of reported cases of AIDS for emergency services and to all States for improved care and support services and early intervention services.

Safe sex: In the context of HIV infection, sexual activity conducted in such a way that there is no risk of transmission or acquisition of the infection (e.g., having a single sexual partner who is not infected with HIV).

Safer sex: Sexual activity conducted in such a way that transmission of HIV infection is minimized by reducing the exchange of body fluids (e.g., consistent use of condoms, avoiding unprotected anal intercourse).

Secondary care setting: A place where patients are referred for special care (e.g., a community or general hospital).

Sensitivity: The ability of a test to correctly identify an individual who is infected.

Seroconversion: The process by which a person's antibody status changes from negative to positive.

Serologic test: Any of a number of tests that are performed on the clear, liquid portion of blood (serum). Often refers to a test that determines the presence of antibodies to antigens such as viruses.

Seronegative: Having a negative test for antibodies to a substance or organism, such as HIV.

Seropositive: Having a positive test for antibodies to a substance or organism, such as HIV.

Seroreverter: Describes a person whose antibody status has changed from positive to negative. Used to describe perinatally exposed infants who are not truly infected and become HIV antibody negative as they lose maternal HIV antibody.

Side effect: Action or effect of a drug other than that desired. The term usually refers to undesired or negative effects (drug toxicity). Investigational drugs must be evaluated for both immediate and long-term side effects.

Sign: An indication of a disease or disorder that is observed by the health care provider.

Squamous intraepithelial lesion (SIL): Findings in cells revealed by Pap smear that indicate changes requiring further evaluation.

Specificity: The ability of a test to correctly identify an individual who is not infected.

Stomatitis: Any of numerous inflammatory diseases of the mouth having various causes (e.g., mechanical trauma, irritants, allergy, vitamin deficiency, infection).

Surrogate markers: Levels of cells or proteins that indirectly indicate HIV activity. CD4 cell counts are surrogate markers of the progression of HIV disease.

Symptom: Any perceptible, subjective change in the body or its functions that indicates disease or phases of disease, as reported by the patient. Should be distinguished from a sign.

Syndrome: A group of symptoms and diseases that together are characteristic of a specific condition.

Syphilis: Infection caused by *T. pallidum* that, if left untreated, can cause chronic infection of multiple organ sites, including the central nervous system. When untreated in pregnant women, can result in a life-threatening congenital infection in the newborn.

Teratogenicity: The ability to cause malformations in a fetus.

Thrush: Oral candidiasis; infection of the mouth or pharynx with the yeast candida. Frequently occurs in persons with a severely damaged immune system; may appear as discrete or confluent white patches on the mucous membranes.

Treatment investigational new drug (IND): Application for the FDA's authorization to use an investigational drug that appears to be safe, and may be effective, in a defined group of patients with serious or life-threatening conditions, and who have no satisfactory alternatives. The purpose is to facilitate availability of promising new drugs as early in the drug development process as possible.

Treponema pallidum: The micro-organism that causes syphilis; sometimes referred to as a spirochete because of its shape.

Trimethoprim-sulfamethoxazole (TMP-SMX): A first-line combination drug for PCP prophylaxis and treatment. Possible side effects include rash, pruritus, cytopenia, liver abnormalities, and gastrointestinal upset.

Tuberculin unit (TU): Term used to describe doses of purified protein derivative.

Tuberculosis: Disease, usually of the lung, caused by the organism *M. tuberculosis.*

Vaccine: A substance that contains antigenic components of an infectious organism. Vaccines stimulate an immune response and may protect or modify subsequent infection by that organism.

Venereal Disease Research Laboratories (VDRL) test: A screening test for syphilis developed at the Venereal Disease Research Laboratories.

Western blot (WB): A test for the presence of antibodies to multiple antigens of HIV; used to confirm HIV infection following a positive ELISA test. The Western Blot displays antibodies to specific HIV viral proteins in a separate, well-defined band. A positive result shows stripes at the locations for two or more viral proteins. A negative result is blank at these locations.

Zalcitabine (ddC; trade name HIVID; also called dideoxycytidine): One of three FDA-approved nucleoside analog drugs that inhibits the reverse transcriptase enzyme of HIV. Its major limiting toxicity is peripheral neuropathy. It has the advantage of being 10 percent more potent than ZDV and has been used in combination therapy with ZDV in patients with advanced disease.

Biosketches: Early HIV Infection Guideline Panel Members

Bruce D. Agins, MD
New York State Department of Health
Dr. Agins is the Assistant Medical Director, AIDS Institute, New York State Department of Health. Dr. Agins serves on a number of professional committees including the Professional Standards Review Council of America, New York State Department of Health and the Medical Advisory Panel, and the AIDS Unit, New York State Department of Substance Abuse Services.

Kay A. Bauman, MD, MPH
Wahiawa General Hospital
Dr. Bauman is an Associate Professor in the Department of Family Practice at the University of Hawaii School of Medicine. She is involved in HIV/AIDS professional education. Formerly, she directed the Arizona AIDS Project for 6 years, receiving funding from the Health Resources and Services Administration and the National Institute of Mental Health for HIV education of health care professionals. She is also active in the care of HIV-infected patients.

Carol L. Brosgart, MD
Alta Bates Medical Center
Dr. Brosgart is trained in pediatrics and preventive medicine and has been caring for patients with HIV disease since 1981. Dr. Brosgart is a member of the clinical faculty at the Schools of Medicine, University of California, San Francisco and Berkeley. She chairs the Scientific Advisory Board of the Community Consortium, an organization of over 300 San Francisco Bay Area HIV providers; is co-chair of the Opportunistic Infections Interest Group of the Community Programs for Clinical Research on AIDS (CPCRA) of the National Institute of Allergy and Infectious Diseases, National Institutes of Health; and is a founding member of the Bay Area Research Consortium on Women and AIDS (BARCWA).

Gina M. Brown, M.D.
Columbia Presbyterian Medical Center
Dr. Brown, who specializes in maternal and fetal medicine, is a Fellow in Critical Care at Columbia Presbyterian Medical Center in New York. Previously, she was a Fellow at the HIV Center at Columbia Presbyterian. Dr. Brown is a member of the AIDS Clinical Advisory Panel of the New York State AIDS Institute.

155

Jaime Geaga, PA-C, MPH
Filipino Task Force on AIDS

Mr. Geaga is a certified Physician Assistant with a masters degree in Health Policy and Administration. He worked for 6 years at Children's Hospital of San Francisco, conducting HIV research and clinical trials. He is a member of the National Executive Board of the National Minority AIDS Council (NMAC). He was the founder of the Filipino Task Force on AIDS which he established in 1988 and was its Executive Director through early 1993. As a person who is HIV-infected, he participated in the HIV guideline panel both as a practitioner and a consumer.

Wafaa El-Sadr, MD, MPH, *Co-Chair*
Harlem Hospital Center

Dr. El-Sadr is the Chief of Infectious Disease at Harlem Hospital, NY, and an Associate Professor of Clinical Medicine at Columbia University College of Physicians and Surgeons. She is also principal investigator of the Harlem AIDS Treatment Group, one of the Community Programs for Clinical Research on AIDS (CPCRA). She has established several clinical, research, and outreach programs primarily focused on HIV infection and tuberculosis. She has published on issues related to recruitment of minorities in clinical trials, women with HIV, pneumocystis, and tuberculosis.

Deborah Greenspan, BDS, Dsc, ScD
University of California, San Francisco

Dr. Greenspan is currently Clinical Professor of Oral Medicine in the Department of Stomatology at the University of California, San Francisco; Chair of the Task Force on Infection Control for the School of Dentistry; and Clinical Director of the Oral AIDS Center. In 1989, she was given the Samuel Charles Miller Award by the American Academy of Oral Medicine. She also was the recipient of an award from the Assistant Secretary for Health for her contributions to work on the AIDS epidemic. In 1993, she was elected to be a fellow of the American Academy of Sciences.

Karen Hein, MD, BMS
Albert Einstein College of Medicine

Dr. Hein, an expert in adolescent medicine for 20 years, founded the Nation's first program focusing on the impact of the HIV epidemic on adolescents. She is President of the Society for Adolescent Medicine (1992-93) and was the recipient of an Assistant Secretary for Health award for an outstanding physician contribution to the AIDS epidemic in 1989. She has written extensively on issues affecting adolescents, particularly high-risk youth.

William L. Holzemer, PhD, RN
University of California, San Francisco

Dr. Holzemer serves as the Director of the Center for HIV/AIDS Clinical Training and Research in Nursing at the School of Nursing, University of California, San Francisco. His research focuses on the quality of nursing care for people living with HIV/AIDS in hospital and home care settings. He chairs the American Academy of Nursing's Expert Panel on HIV/AIDS.

Rudolph E. Jackson, MD
Morehouse School of Medicine

Dr. Jackson is the Director of the Association of Minority Health Professions Schools AIDS Research Consortium, Morehouse School of Medicine, and Director of the Zambian HIV/AIDS Prevention Program, US Agency for International Development. He was previously Professor and Chairman of the Department of Pediatrics, Meharry Medical College in Nashville. Dr. Jackson has served on numerous professional committees ranging from the National Arthritis, Metabolism, and Digestive Diseases Advisory Council to the Georgia State Task Force on Sickle Cell Disease and has received many awards and honors, including the L.W. Diggs Meritorious Service Award, the Julia Davis Humanitarian Award, the Young Americans Keystone Club Award, and the Sickle Cell Anemia Award.

Michael K. Lindsay, MD, MPH
Grady Memorial Hospital

Dr. Lindsay is a specialist in high-risk obstetrics at Grady Memorial Hospital and Associate Professor of Obstetrics and Gynecology at Emory University. He was instrumental in instituting the Kinst Routine Voluntary Antepartum HIV Screening Program in the United States. Data from this surveillance program have helped advance our understanding of the epidemiology of HIV infection in pregnancy.

Harvey J. Makadon, MD
Harvard Medical School

Dr. Makadon is the Associate Director, Division of General Medicine and Primary Care, and the Medical Director of Ambulatory Services at Beth Israel Hospital, Boston, MA. He is also an Assistant Professor of Medicine at Harvard Medical School. He has been involved in developing the primary care-based AIDS program at Beth Israel. He was the founder and has been the Executive Director and Chair of the Steering Committee of the Boston AIDS Consortium. He is currently Chair of the AIDS Task Force of the Society of General Internal Medicine and the AIDS Task Force of the Conference of Boston Teaching Hospitals.

Martha W. Moon, MS, RN
San Francisco, CA
Martha Moon is the former Clinical Director of the Fenway Community Health Center in Boston, MA. In this role, she was responsible for the development and implementation of the Outpatient HIV Treatment Center and was Manager of the Research Department. Her current interests include risk factors for HIV in runaway and homeless adolescents and access to HIV clinical trials for adolescents.

James M. Oleske, MD, MPH, *Co-Chair*
New Jersey Medical School
Dr. Oleske is Francois-Xavier Bagnoud Professor of Pediatrics and Director, Division of Allergy, Immunology, and Infectious Diseases of the University of Medicine and Dentistry of New Jersey. He is also Medical Director of the Children's Hospital AIDS Program (CHAP) of New Jersey, one of the nation's largest treatment centers for childhood AIDS.

Claire Rappoport, MS
San Francisco General Hospital
Ms. Rappoport is the Project Manager of the Community Provider AIDS Training Project at the University of California, San Francisco. She is a member of the Advisory Forum of the Community Consortium, a clinical trials group. She also serves on the Advisory Board of the California Nurses Association's Women at Risk: HIV/AIDS Training for Care Providers Program and as a speaker for the San Francisco Department of Public Health's Wedge Program. She has served on the Mayor's San Francisco HIV Health Services Planning Council and the Advisory Board of the Women's AIDS Network and as a consultant to the UCSF AIDS Health Project's Positive Being Positive peer support program.

Gwendolyn B. Scott, MD
University of Miami School of Medicine
Dr. Scott is a Professor of Pediatrics and the Director of the Division of Pediatric Infectious Diseases and Immunology at the University of Miami School of Medicine. She was among the first to describe HIV infection in children and has been actively involved in the clinical care and treatment of children with HIV infection since 1981. She has served as consultant to the National Institutes of Health, the Centers for Disease Control and Prevention, and the World Health Organization on issues related to pediatric AIDS and is the Chairman of the American Academy of Pediatrics Committee on AIDS.

Walter W. Shervington, MD
Louisiana Department of Health and Hospitals
Dr. Shervington is Assistant Secretary, Office of Mental Health, Louisiana Department of Health and Hospitals. He is also Associate Professor of Psychiatry at Louisiana State University School of Medicine and Director of Neuropsychosocial Services, HIV Outpatient Program at Charity Hospital and is on the faculty of the Delta Region AIDS Education and Training Center, Louisiana State University Medical School and Tulane University School of Public Health and Tropical Medicine. Dr. Shervington is a Fellow of the American Psychiatric Association.

Lawrence C. Shulman, MSW, ACSW
Sociomedical Resource Associates
Mr. Shulman is a partner in a health care consulting firm, specializing in organizational and administrative redesign, program and services development and evaluation, case management, and grant development. His social work and administrative experience is in the areas of HIV/AIDS, substance abuse, maternal and child health, and gerontology. Mr. Shulman was instrumental in the development of case management standards for the NY State Department of Health/AIDS Institute Designated AIDS Centers as well as integrated health/social work services programs for at-risk mothers and children.

Constance B. Wofsy, MD, MA
University of California, San Francisco
Dr. Wofsy is Professor of Clinical Medicine at the University of California, San Francisco. She is Co-Director, AIDS Activities Division; Interim Director, AIDS Clinic, San Francisco General Hospital; and Associate Chief of the Infectious Diseases Division (Acting Chief, 1991) at San Francisco General Hospital. In addition to being the Director of APEX (AIDS Provider Education and Experience, 1976-present), she is the Founding Chair of the Women's Health Committee of the ACTG (1991-1993) and serves as well on the AIDS Program Advisory Committee for NIH.

Contributors[1]

Panel Staff

Robin Flam, DrPH
Project Coordinator
Harlem Hospital Center
New York, NY

Marie Stallings
New Jersey Medical School
Newark, NJ

David Steven Rappoport
Harlem Hospital Center
New York, NY

E. Niki Warin
Harlem Hospital Center
New York, NY

Myriam Sudit, PhD
New Jersey Medical School
Newark, NJ

Consultants

Robert F. Nease, Jr, PhD
Methodologist
Dartmouth Medical School
Hanover, NH

Douglas K. Owens, MD
Methodologist
Palo Alto VA Medical Center
Palo Alto, CA

Lawrence Bartlett, PhD
Health Policy Analyst
Health Systems Research, Inc.
Washington, DC

Peer Reviewers

Donald Abrams, MD
Associate Professor of Clinical
Medicine
San Fransisco General Hospital
San Francisco, CA

Jean R. Anderson, MD
Department of Obstetrics/
Gynecology
John Hopkins Hospital
Baltimore, MD

Arthur Ashe (Deceased)
Consumer
New York, NY

Charles N. Aswad, MD
Physician Service Associates
Binghamton, NY

Arlene Bardequez, MD
Department of Obstetrics/
Gynecology/Perinatology
University of Medicine and
Dentistry of New Jersey
Newark, NJ

Mary Boland, RN
Director, CHAP Program
Children's Hospital of New Jersey
Newark, NJ

---

[1] Being listed as a contributor does not necessarily imply endorsement of the guideline.

161

Richard Brown, MD
Director
Ambulatory Pediatrics and
Adolescent Medicine
San Francisco General Hospital
San Francisco, CA

William Caspe, MD
Director, Department of Pediatrics
Bronx-Lebanon Hospital
New York, NY

Ronnie Davidson, EdD
Director, Research and Education
The Academy of Medicine
Lawrenceville, NJ

Larry D'Angelo, MD
Chairman, Department of
Adolescent and Young
Adult Medicine
Children's National Medical
Center
Washington, DC

Dorothy Friedberg, MD
Department of Ophthalmology
New York University Medical
Center
New York, NY

Aaron Glatt, MD
Chief, Division of Infectious
Diseases
Catholic Medical Center of
Brooklyn and Queens
New York, NY

Lewis Goldfrank, MD
Emergency Medicine
Bellevue Hospital Center
New York, NY

Sandra Hernandez, MD
Director, AIDS Office
San Francisco Department of
Public Health
San Francisco, CA

Washington Hill, MD
Professor and Chairman, Depart-
ment of Obstetrics/Gynecology
Meharry Medical College
Nashville, TN

Steve Lew
Gay Asian Pacific Alliance Co.
HIV Project
San Francisco, CA

Mary C. Magee, RN
San Francisco, CA

Gloria Maki
Case Manager, New York State
Department of Health
AIDS Institute
New York, NY

Carola Marte, MD
Beth Israel Medical Center
New York, NY

Howard Minkoff, MD
Professor of Obstetrics/
Gynecology
SUNY Downstate Health Science
New York, NY

Anthony B. Minnefor, MD
Chairman, Pediatrics
St. Barnabas Medical Center
Livingston, NJ

Mark D. Mintz, MD
Assistant Professor of
Neurosciences and Pediatrics
University of Medicine and
Dentistry of New Jersey
Newark, NJ

Barry Moore, MSW
Social Work Services
University Hospital
Newark, NJ

Paul Moore, MSW
Assistant Vice-President
Professional Services and
Affiliations
New York City Health and
Hospital Corporation
New York, NY

Julie Graves Moy, MD, MPH
Clinical Assistant Professor
Department of Family Medicine
Baylor College of Medicine
Houston, TX

Daniel Musher, MD
Chief, Infectious Disease Section
Veterans Affairs Medical Center
Houston, TX

Joan Phelan, DDS
Columbia Presbyterian
Medical Center
New York, NY

David Potts, MD
Director, Internal Medicine
Residency Program
Greenville Memorial Medical
Center
Greenville, SC

Michael Reyes, MD
Medical Director
Western Area AIDS Education
San Francisco, CA

Richard G. Roberts, MD, JD
Associate Professor
Department of Family Medicine
and Practice
University of Wisconsin
Medical School
Madison, WI

Polly Ross, MD
Blue Ridge Health Center
Henderson, NC

Benjamin Rush, MD
Department of Surgery
New Jersey Medical School
Newark, NJ

Edward Telzak, MD
Chief, Infectious Diseases
Bronx Lebanon Hospital
New York, NY

Anita Vaughn, MD
Newark, NJ

Patricia Whitley-Williams, MD
Morehouse School of Medicine
Department of Pediatrics
Nashville, TN

Reggie Williams
National Task Force on AIDS
Prevention
San Francisco, CA

Thomas Wright, MD
Department of Pathology
Columbia Presbyterian
Medical Center
New York, NY

Note: The Panel also wishes to acknowledge the anonymous clinician and patient feasibility reviewers, as well as those HIV-positive persons and parents or caretakers of HIV-positive children who took part in focus group testing of the two consumer guides.

163

Appendix A. Algorithms

Algorithm 1. Selected Elements of the Initial and Ongoing Evaluation of Adults with Early HIV Infection

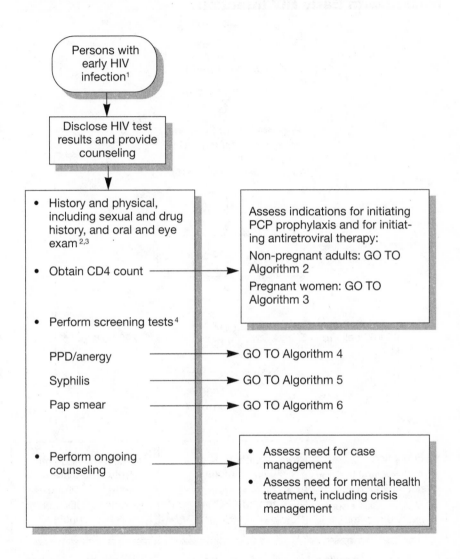

[1] Provider should review and evaluate the adequacy of HIV diagnostic tests.

[2] Appropriate immunizations should be provided (this topic was not reviewed by the HIV panel).

[3] Schedule followup appropriate for patient's condition.

[4] Many other screening tests were not reviewed by this panel, including toxoplasmosis, hepatitis serology, and routine laboratory tests.

Note: The algorithm presents recommendations only for the items reviewed by the HIV panel.

Algorithm 2. Evaluation for Initiation of Antiretroviral Therapy and PCP Prophylaxis; Men and Nonpregnant Women with Early HIV Infection

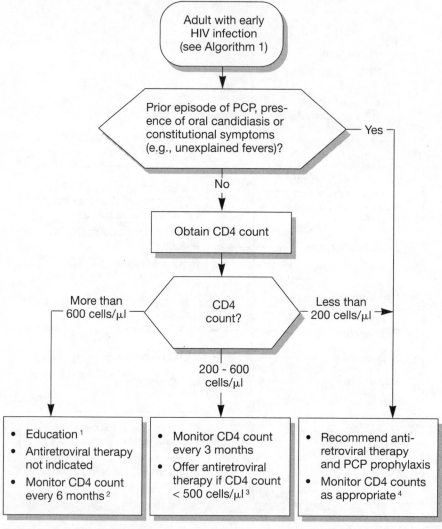

[1] Education should include a discussion of enrollment into relevant investigational drug trials for asymptomatic persons.

[2] If CD4 count has shown great variability or is rapidly declining, repeat the CD4 within 3 months.

[3] If patient develops symptoms, recommend antiretroviral therapy.

[4] If CD4 count < 200 cells/ml, continued monitoring of CD4 count may be needed to determine eligibility for clinical trials, and prophylaxis for opportunistic infections other than PCP and to guide antiretroviral therapy.

Note: The algorithm presents recommendations only for the items reviewed by the HIV panel.

Algorithm 3. Evaluation for Initiation of Antiretroviral Therapy and PCP Prophylaxis; Pregnant Women with Early HIV Infection

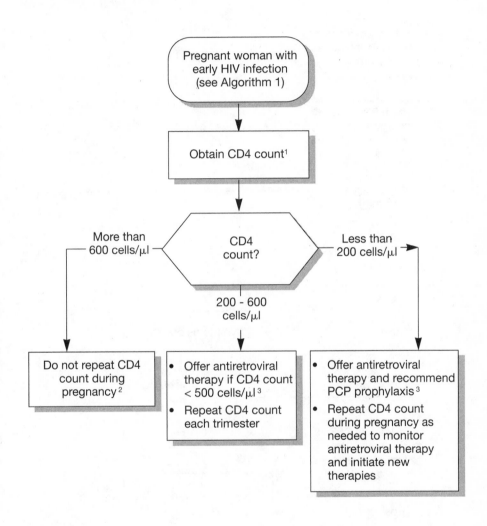

[1] CD4 count should be obtained on presentation for prenatal care; women who have received no prenatal care should have CD4 counts taken at delivery.

[2] Unless indicated by the presence of clinical symptoms.

[3] The possible benefits and risks of antiretroviral therapy to both mother and fetus should be discussed fully with the patient.

Note: The algorithm presents recommendations only for the items reviewed by the HIV panel.

Algorithm 4. Evaluation for *Mycobacterium tuberculosis* Infection in Adults and Adolescents with Early HIV Infection

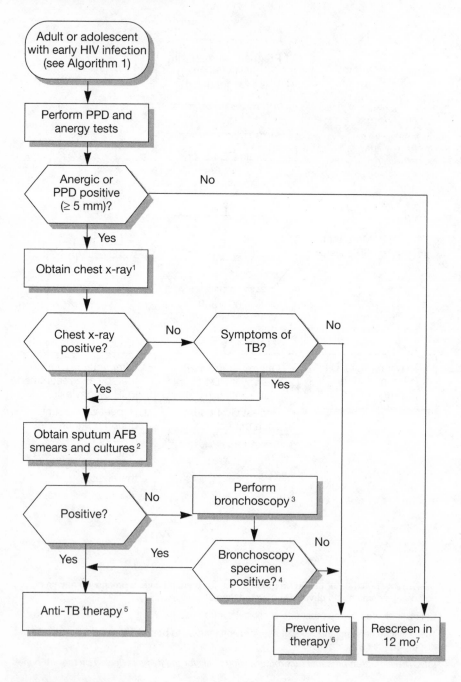

[1] Chest x-ray can be performed, using a lead apron shield, after the first trimester in pregnant women asymptomatic for TB or at any stage of pregnancy in women symptomatic for TB.

[2] At least three sputum smears and cultures should be obtained.

[3] If there is no other etiology for the abnormal chest x-ray.

[4] Both AFB smears and cultures should be obtained at bronchoscopy.

[5] Anti-TB therapy should be guided by local susceptibility patterns and modified appropriately when isolated susceptibilities become available.

[6] Preventive therapy is indicated for PPD-positive patients and should be strongly considered for anergic patients who are known contacts of patients with tuberculosis and for anergic patients belonging to groups in which the prevalence of tuberculosis is at least 10% (e.g., injection drug users, prisoners, homeless persons, persons in congregate housing, migrant laborers, and persons born in foreign countries with high rates of TB).

[7] Individuals who reside in settings where TB prevalence is high should be retested in 6 months; individuals who are exposed acutely to others with suspected or confirmed TB should be retested in 3 months; anergic individuals need not be retested, except in special circumstances.

Note: The algorithm presents recommendations only for the items reviewed by the HIV panel.

Algorithm 5. Evaluation for Syphilis in Adults and Sexually Active Adolescents with Early HIV Infection

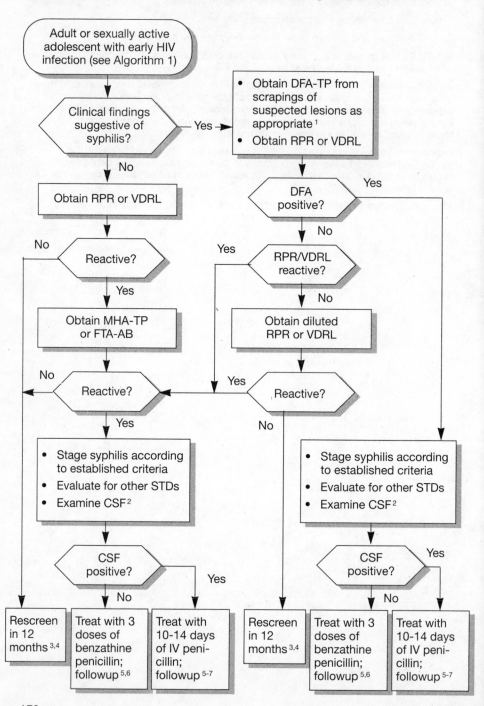

[1] If dark-field exam cannot be performed and primary syphilis is suspected, empiric treatment should be instituted.

[2] Treatment for neurosyphilis recommended if the CSF cannot be evaluated (See *Guideline for Evaluation and Management of Early HIV Infection* for recommended followup).

[3] Or after exposure to or diagnosis of any sexually transmitted disease.

[4] Pregnant women should be screened for syphilis at entry to prenatal care, during the third trimester, or at delivery.

[5] See *Guideline for Evaluation and Management of Early HIV Infection* for recommended followup.

[6] For issues specific to pregnant women, see Guideline for Evaluation and Management of Early HIV Infection for recommended followup.

[7] Alternative treatments include 10 days of IM procaine penicillin or 10-14 days of 1-2 g of IM ceftriaxome.

Note: The algorithm presents recommendations only for the items reviewed by the HIV panel.

Algorithm 6. Pap Smears in Women with Early HIV Infection

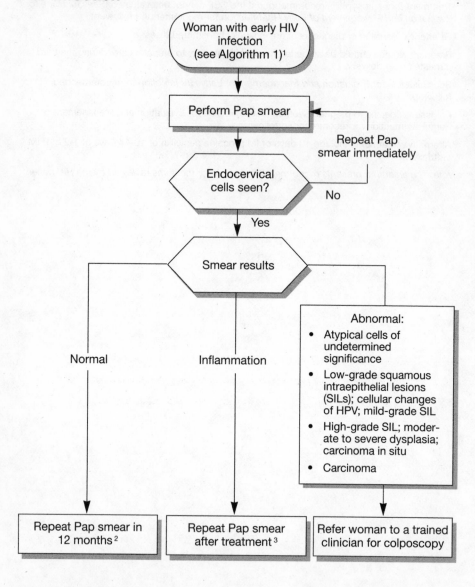

Woman with early HIV infection (see Algorithm 1)[1]

Perform Pap smear

Endocervical cells seen?

Repeat Pap smear immediately

No

Yes

Smear results

Normal

Inflammation

Abnormal:
- Atypical cells of undetermined significance
- Low-grade squamous intraepithelial lesions (SILs); cellular changes of HPV; mild-grade SIL
- High-grade SIL; moderate to severe dysplasia; carcinoma in situ
- Carcinoma

Repeat Pap smear in 12 months[2]

Repeat Pap smear after treatment[3]

Refer woman to a trained clinician for colposcopy

[1] Pap smears should be performed at entry to prenatal care for pregnant women and prior to discharge for women who present for delivery without prenatal care.

[2] HIV-infected women with a history of human papilloma virus (HPV) or with previous Pap smears showing squamous intraepithelial lesions should have their Pap smears repeated every 6 months.

[3] Treatment should be guided by diagnosis of the cause of inflammation.

Note: The algorithm presents recommendations only for the items reviewed by the HIV panel.

Algorithm 7: Evaluation for Initiation of Antiretroviral Therapy and PCP Prophylaxis; Infants and Children with Early HIV Infection

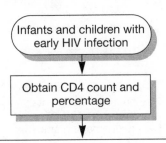

Infants and children with early HIV infection

↓

Obtain CD4 count and percentage

↓

- Initiate antiretroviral therapy as indicated by either CD4 count (Table A) or CD4 percentage (Table B)
- Initiate PCP prophylaxis as indicated by either CD4 count (Figure A) or CD4 percentage (Figure B)[1]
- Infants and children receiving neither antiretroviral therapy nor PCP prophylaxis should have their CD4 counts and percentages monitored[2]

Figure A

Age	CD4 count (cells/ml) 200 300 500 750 1000 1500 1750
<12 mo[1]	
12–24 mo[2]	
2–6 yr[2]	
≥6 yr[2]	

▓ Initiate PCP prophylaxis
■ Initiate antiretroviral therapy

Figure B

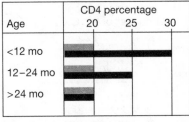

Age	CD4 percentage 20 25 30
<12 mo	
12–24 mo	
>24 mo	

▓ Initiate PCP prophylaxis
■ Initiate antiretroviral therapy

Source: Figure A adapted from Centers for Disease Control, 1991

[1] Patients with prior episode of PCP should receive PCP prophylaxis regardless of CD4 count and percentage.

[2] Obtain CD4 count and percentage at 1 month of age, 3 months of age, and then at 3 month intervals through 24 months of age; thereafter obtain CD4 count and percentage every 6 months, unless values reach an age-related threshold where testing should be repeated monthly.

Note: The algorithm presents recommendations only for the items reviewed by the HIV panel.

Algorithm 8. Neurologic Evaluation of Infants and Children with Early HIV Infection

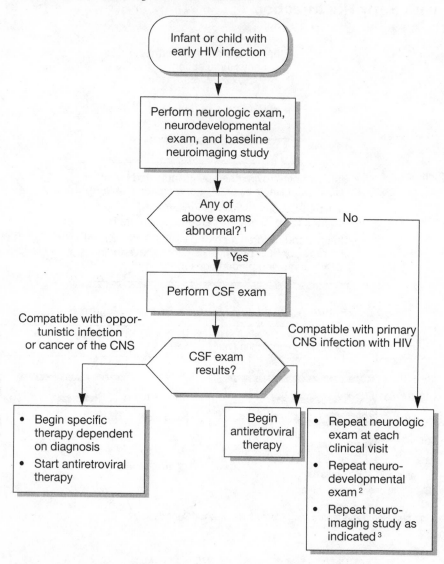

[1] Abnormal exam is defined as focal pathology, obstructive lesion, atypical CNS manifestations, or evidence of progressive neurologic disease (see Guideline for Evaluation and Management of Early HIV Infection).

[2] Neurodevelopmental exams should be performed at 3 month intervals up to 24 months of age, then every 6 months thereafter.

[3] Neuroimaging studies should be performed if CNS symptoms occur; such studies should be performed in conjunction with CSF analysis.

Note: The algorithm presents recommendations only for the items reviewed by the HIV panel.

Appendix B. Drug Dosing Information

Appendix B-1. Drug dosage[1] and adverse effects; *Pneumocystis carinii* pneumonia prophylaxis[2]

Medication	Dosage Adult/Tanner stage IV and V adolescents[3]
Trimethoprim-Sulfamethoxazole (TMP-SMX) Bactrim® Septra® Formulations: Single-strength tablet: 80 mg TMP 400 mg SMX Double-strength tablet: 160 mg TMP 800 mg SMX Pediatric suspension: (per 5 ml) 40 mg TMP 200 mg SMX	Most commonly used regimens: one double-strength tablet taken orally three times per week on alternate days or daily 7 days per week
Pentamidine Isethionate NebuPent® 300 mg The vial must be dissolved in 6 ml sterile water and used with Respirguard® nebulizer	Aerosolized pentamidine (AP) (NebuPent®) is given as single 300 mg (one vial) dose every 4 weeks. Nebulized dose given over 30-45 min at a flow rate of 5-9 liters/min from a 40-50 lb per square inch air or oxygen source Alternative: if a Fisons ultrasonic nebulizer is used, dose of pentamidine is 60 mg given every 2 weeks after a loading dose of five treatments given over 2 weeks
Dapsone Formulation: 25 and 100 mg tablets	50-100 mg total daily oral dose divided into two doses or administered as a single daily dose given 2-7 times per week daily dose given 7 days per week

[1] Contains only drugs discussed or recommended in the *Clinical Practice Guideline for Evaluation and Management of Early HIV Infection.* Not all drugs or combinations of drugs used in the care of HIV-infected individuals are included.

[2] Dosage schedules and recommendations for use are based on review of literature or expert consensus and may not have approval of the Food and Drug Administration (FDA) for indications noted. Information included in this guideline may not represent FDA approval or FDA-approved labeling for the particular products or indications in question. Specifically, the terms "safe" and "effective" may not be synonymous with the FDA-defined legal standard for product approval.

Dosage Infants/children/ Tanner stage I and II adolescents [3]	Adverse effects [4]
150 mg/m^2 TMP 750 mg/m^2 SMX Total oral daily dose given 3 times/week Can be divided into two doses or administered as a single daily dose and given on 3 consecutive or 3 alternate days per week This same oral daily dose divided into 2 doses can be given 7 days per week	Drug allergy: Skin rash Steven-Johnson syndrome Fever Arthralgia Toxic epidermal necrolysis Hematologic: Anemia Neutropenia Thrombocytopenia Gastrointestinal: Elevation of serum transaminase Nausea Vomiting Anorexia Fulminant hepatic necrosis (rare)
Children over 5 yr can receive same inhalation dose as adults	Pulmonary: Bronchospasm with cough Pneumothorax Other: Extrapulmonary *P. carinii* infection Increased risk of environmental transmission of *M. tuberculosis*
1 mg/kg administered orally as a single daily dose given 7 days per week	Hematologic: Agranulocytosis Aplastic anemia Hemolytic anemia in G6PD deficiency Methemoglobinemia Cutaneous reactions: Bullous and exfoliative dermatitis Erythema nodosum Erythema multiforme Peripheral neuropathy Gastrointestinal: Nausea Vomiting

[3] For adolescents who are Tanner stage I or II, pediatric dose schedules should be followed. Adult doses should be used for adolescents who are Tanner stage IV or V. Tanner stage III adolescents should have dose individualized, recognizing that this is the stage of most rapid growth.

[4] For a complete list of adverse reactions to these drugs, consult the *Physicians' Desk Reference* (Medical Economics Data, Montvale, NJ, 1993) or the drug's package insert.

Appendix B-2. Drug[1] dosage and adverse effects; Antiretroviral therapy[2]

Medication	Dosage Adult/Tanner stage IV and V adolescents[3]	Dosage Infants/children/ Tanner stage I and II adolescents[3]	Adverse effects[4]
Zidovudine (ZDV) formerly azidothymidine (AZT) Retrovir® Formulation: 100 mg capsules Pediatric syrup 50 mg/5 ml	100 mg/dose administered orally every 4 hours or 5 doses given 7 days/week	180 mg/m² dose administered orally every 6 hours given 7 days/week	Granulocytopenia Anemia Nausea Headache Confusion Myositis Anorexia Hepatitis Seizures Nail discoloration
Didanosine (ddI) (dideoxyinosine) Videx® Formulation: 25, 50, 100, 150 mg tablets Pediatric powder for oral solution 10 mg/ml	Patients under 45 kg: 100 mg/dose orally given every 12 hours 7 days/week Patients over 45 kg: 200 mg/dose administered orally every 12 hours given 7 days/week (Tablet should be chewed and taken on an empty stomach)	200 mg/m²/day administered orally every 12 hours given 7 days per week	Pancreatitis, potentially fatal Peripheral neuropathy Peripheral retinal atrophy (in children only) Nausea Diarrhea Confusion Seizures
Zalcitabine (ddC) (dideoxycitidine) Formulation: 0.375 mg tablets 0.750 mg tablets Pediatric 0.1 mg/ml syrup	Patients under 45 kg: 0.375 mg/dose administered orally every 8 hours given 7 days/week Patients over 45 kg: 0.750 mg dose administered orally every 8 hours given 7 days/week	0.005-0.01 mg/kg/ dose administered orally every 8 hours given 7 days/week	Aphthous ulcers Esophageal ulcers Peripheral neuropathy Stomatitis Cutaneous eruptions Thrombocytopenia Pancreatitis

[1] Contains only drugs discussed or recommended in the *Clinical Practice Guideline for Evaluation and Management of Early HIV Infection.* Not all drugs or combinations of drugs used in the care of HIV-infected individuals are included.

[2] Dosage schedules and recommendations for use are based on review of literature or expert consensus and may not have approval of the Food and Drug Administration (FDA) for indications noted. Information included in this guideline may not represent FDA approval or FDA-approved labeling for the particular products or indications in question. Specifically, the terms "safe" and "effective" may not be synonymous with the FDA-defined legal standard for product approval.

[3] For adolescents who are Tanner stage I or II, pediatric dose schedules should be followed. Adult doses should be used for adolescents who are Tanner stage IV or V. Tanner stage III adolescents should have dose individualized, recognizing that this is the stage of most rapid growth.

[4] For a complete list of adverse reactions to these drugs, consult the *Physicians' Desk Reference* (Medical Economics Data, Montvale, NJ, 1993) or the drug's package insert.

Appendix B-3. Drug[1] dosage and adverse effects; Preventive therapy (chemoprophylaxis) for *Mycobacterium tuberculosis*[2]

Medication	Dosage: Adult/Tanner stage IV and V adolescents[3]	Dosage: Infants/children/ Tanner stage I and II adolescents[3]	Adverse effects[4]
Isoniazid INHR Nydrazid® Formulation: 50 mg, 100 mg, 300 mg tablets 1 gram vial Syrup 50 mg/5 ml	300 mg administered orally as a single daily dose given 7 days/wk for 12 mo or 900 mg administered orally as a single daily dose given 2 days/week for 12 mo	10-15 mg/kg/day (max 300 mg/day) administered orally as a single daily dose given 7 days/wk for 12 mo	Gastrointestinal: Hepatotoxicity (rare in children) Nausea, vomiting, anorexia Neurologic: Peripheral neuropathy Neuritis, fatigue Weakness Hematologic: Agranulocytosis Hemolytic and aplastic anemia Thrombocytopenia Eosinophilia Drug Allergy: Skin rash Fever Lymphadenopathy and vasculitis (SLE-like syndrome)

[1] Contains only drugs discussed or recommended in the *Clinical Practice Guideline for Evaluation and Management of Early HIV Infection.* Not all drugs or combinations of drugs used in the care of HIV-infected individuals are included.

[2] Dosage schedules and recommendations for use are based on review of literature or expert consensus and may not have approval of the Food and Drug Administration (FDA) for indications noted. Information included in this guideline may not represent FDA approval or FDA-approved labeling for the particular products or indications in question. Specifically, the terms "safe" and "effective" may not be synonymous with the FDA-defined legal standard for product approval.

[3] For adolescents who are Tanner stage I or II, pediatric dose schedules should be followed. Adult doses should be used for adolescents who are Tanner stage IV or V. Tanner stage III adolescents should have dose individualized, recognizing that this is the stage of most rapid growth.

[4] For a complete list of adverse reactions to these drugs, consult the *Physicians' Desk Reference* (Medical Economics Data, Montvale, NJ, 1993) or the drug's package insert.

Appendix C

C-1. Sources of HIV information

General information:

English: (800) 342-AIDS (2437)
Spanish: (800) 344-7432
TDD Service for the Deaf: (800) 243-7889

General information for health care providers:

HIV Telephone Consultation Service: (800) 933-3413

State hotlines:

For information about HIV-specific resources and counseling and testing services, call your State AIDS hotline:

Alabama . . . . (800) 228-0469
Alaska . . . . (800) 478-2437
Arizona . . . . (800) 548-4695
Arkansas . . . . (800) 661-2133
California (No.) . . . . (800) 367-2437
California (So.) . . . . (800) 922-2437
Colorado . . . . (800) 252-2437
Connecticut . . . . (800) 342-2437
Delaware . . . . (800) 422-0429
District of Columbia . . . . (800) 332-2437
Florida . . . . (800) 352-2437
Georgia . . . . (800) 551-2728
Hawaii . . . . (800) 922-1313
Idaho . . . . (800) 345-2277
Illinois . . . . (800) 243-2437
Indiana . . . . (800) 848-2437
Iowa . . . . (800) 445-2437
Kansas . . . . (800) 232-0040
Kentucky . . . . (800) 654-2437
Louisiana . . . . (800) 922-4379
Maine . . . . (800) 851-2437
Maryland . . . . (800) 638-6252
Massachusetts . . . . (800) 235-2331
Michigan . . . . (800) 827-2437
Minnesota . . . . (800) 248-2437
Mississippi . . . . (800) 537-0851
Missouri . . . . (800) 533-2437
Montana . . . . (800) 233-6668
Nebraska . . . . (800) 782-2437
Nevada . . . . (800) 842-2437
New Hampshire . . . . (800) 324-2437

New Jersey...(800) 624-2377
New Mexico ....(800) 545-2437
New York..(800) 541-2437
North Carolina ....(800) 733-7301
North Dakota..(800) 472-2180
Ohio ....(800) 332-2437
Oklahoma ....(800) 535-2437
Oregon...(800) 777-2437
Pennsylvania..(800) 662-6080
Puerto Rico..(800) 765-1010
Rhode Island ....(800) 726-3010
South Carolina..(800) 322-2437
South Dakota..(800) 592-1861
Tennessee...(800) 525-2437
Texas..(800) 299-2437
Utah ....(800) 366-2437
Vermont ....(800) 882-2437
Virginia ....(800) 533-4148
Virgin Islands...(800) 773-2437
Washington ....(800) 272-2437
West Virginia ....(800) 642-8244
Wisconsin...(800) 334-2437
Wyoming ....(800) 327-3577

For HIV/AIDS treatment information, call:

The American Foundation
 for AIDS Research ....(800) 39AMFAR (392-6327)

AIDS Treatment Data Network ....(212) 268-4196

AIDS Treatment News...................(800) TREAT 1-2 (873-2812)

For information about AIDS/HIV clinical trials conducted by National Institutes of Health and Food and Drug Administration-approved efficacy trials, call:

AIDS Clinical Trials Information
 Service (ACTIS)......................(800) TRIALS-A (874-2572)

To locate a physician, call your local or State Medical Society

For more information about HIV infection, call:

Drug Abuse Hotline...................... (800) 662-HELP (4357)

Pediatric and Pregnancy
 AIDS Hotline .... (212) 430-3333

National Hemophilia Foundation........ (212) 219-8180

Hemophilia and AIDS/HIV Network for Dissemination
 of Information (HANDI).............. (800) 42-HANDI (424-2634)

National Pediatric HIV
 Resource Center .... (800) 362-0071

National Association of People
 with AIDS.............................. (202) 898-0414

Teens Teaching AIDS Prevention Program (TTAPP)
 National Hotline:...................... (800) 234-TEEN (8336)

Note: This is not an all-inclusive list. For other sources of information, contact your State HIV hotline (see preceding list).

C-2. Reporting requirements for human immunodeficiency virus (HIV) infection

By name	Anonymous	Not Required
Alabama	Georgia	Alaska
Arizona	Iowa	California
Arkansas	Kansas	Connecticut
Colorado	Kentucky	Delaware
Idaho	Maine	Florida
Illinois	Montana	Hawaii
Indiana	New Hampshire	Louisiana
Michigan	Oregon	Maryland[2]
Minnesota	Rhode Island	Massachusetts
Mississippi	Texas	Nebraska
Missouri		New Mexico
Nevada		New York
New Jersey[1]		Pennsylvania
North Carolina		Vermont
North Dakota		Washington[2]
Ohio		District of Columbia
Oklahoma		
South Carolina		
South Dakota		
Tennessee[1]		
Utah		
Virginia		
West Virginia		
Wisconsin		
Wyoming		

---

[1] Implementation date, January 1992

[2] Requires reports of symptomatic HIV infection by name.

Note: Current as of March 1, 1993. All States require reporting of acquired immunodeficiency syndrome (AIDS) cases by name at the State/local level.

Index

☆ U.S. GOVERNMENT PRINTING OFFICE:1994-363-769/90664